SupremeHealing

by kac young PhD, ND, DCH, RScM

Published by Marlene Morris Ministries, Inc.

Cover design: Marlene Morris
Internal illustrations: kac young & Marlene Morris
Back Cover photo: Marlene Morris
ISBN: 9781453777954

First Printing July 2010
Second Printing December 2010
Third Printing August 2019

Table of Contents

Dedicated to:

Marlene Morris,
whose healing heart inspires and strengthen all who
know her

Violet Thornbush,
whose healing ways remain vivid in my heart

Lisa Tenzin-Dolma,
whose brilliance, talent, love and friendship inspire me
daily

Gordon Smith (in memoriam)
who encouraged me to be the more than I ever thought
I could be

Acknowledgments

Dr. Serge King for his brilliant melding of today's world with the traditions of the Hawaiian Kahuna and for preserving the ancient ways of healing that can help us all.

Dr. Colleen Kennedy for 6 decades of friendship, her wisdom, and her unfaltering dedication to the education of America.

Dr. John Fitzgerald who heals by just walking into a room.

Dr. Ruth Marie Gibbons who has touched the world and made it better by her love of theater, her brilliance as a thinker and her skill as a teacher.

Dr. Greg Manteuffel the most dedicated, professional and inspiring homeopath I have ever met.

Terah Kathryn Collins who is an inspiration and lives to create more harmony and balance in our world every day.

Jerry Luedders who knows more about healing from the inside out than anyone I know. His dedication to helping people realize their place in Divinity is breathtaking.

Foreword

kac young is, by nature, a true healer. I have seen her at work. I have witnessed her skillful application of the healing processes she describes in this book. And I have experienced first-hand the results of her dedicated work.

She did not decide to become a medical professional, though she is certainly intelligent enough to have accomplished that goal. Instead, throughout her life she has studied a myriad of the world's healing disciplines, both practical and esoteric, and synthesized a model for healing that is based on the marriage of practical knowledge and spiritual principles.

Supreme Healing is not a medical text, nor is it a book to be lightly scanned and set aside. It is a guidebook to healing on many levels. With wit and wisdom, the author takes the reader by the hand and, calling forth the healer within, points the way to the wholeness.

kac is, by nature, a healer. Her point, throughout this book, is that we are all, by nature, healers and that we have within us the energy and the power to overcome any condition. The information in this book is solid, the tools are user friendly, and the processes are dynamic. The only thing that needs to be added is a willingness to consider illness in a new light and to accept your own innate healing powers.

Open the book, open your mind, and you will be on the path to *Supreme Healing*.

Marlene Morris, D.D.

Author's Invitation

I invite you to consider the ideas in this book as a necklace of healing wisdom; ideas that have been collected over time and assembled one jewel at a time until the necklace was complete.

Think of it as gathering your favorite treasures, no matter what they may be, and linking them together, one by one, until they form a continuous circle of knowledge and understanding. The invisible thread of your consciousness strings the healing ideas and concepts on a garland of inspiration which you hold in your mind. Once complete, it is yours to wear permanently; you need never take it off.

The first three chapters of *Supreme Healing* explore the various ways to perceive healing and suggest new paradigms for considering and unraveling the primeval mystery. These pearls of wisdom are the beginning of your collection of insights about that which has stumped science, medicine and healers for centuries.

Chapters Four through Six add more jewels to your collection as they illustrate and define the three steps you can learn and follow to activate your personal healing process. Chapter Seven instructs you in the ultimate power tool: The Act of *Supreme Healing.*

Your healing begins on page one and you will create a personal revolution as you make the journey toward renewed health through an understanding of the spiritual art, the invisible tools and practices of the healer within.

Joyous Healing.

Introduction

What if you were paid to heal? At this moment there are hundreds of companies paying their employees to lose weight and stay healthy. They provide financial incentives for weight loss, and exercise; and they have achieved positive results that include lower health care costs, fewer sick days and increased productivity with more satisfaction and job contentment.[1]

What if someone came along and offered, *"I'll give you $100,000 to heal yourself"* ? What would you do? Would you accept the offer? If you did accept it, how would you set about the task? Would you sit down and make an elaborately detailed plan and follow it? Would you call your friends and family and ask them what you should do? Would you immediately go to your doctor and ask him or her for suggestions and prescriptions? Would you go online and order a bunch of books from Amazon? Would you find a shaman and make an appointment? Would you travel to a foreign country? Would you call in your spirit guides? What would you do? How would you begin the process of healing? And, what exactly do you think healing is?

To help provide considerations to these questions, I wrote this book. I wanted to create a vehicle that would explore the meaning of healing, inspire the process of healing and shed some light on the mystery surrounding healing.

---

[1] http://articles.moneycentral.msn.com/Insurance/InsureYourHealth/GetPaid ToLoseWeight.aspx

No one completely understands healing; it has fascinated the brightest and the most erudite thinkers and philosophers for centuries. No one yet has found the perfect definition or explanation. But there are directions to explore, doors to unlock and visions to behold that can unravel the mysterious intricacies and ultimately transport us from one physical condition into another.

Healing is a fascinating subject and one that we will explore together. After all, there's a huge goal at stake: the quality and the length of our lives.

This book is a beginning. I hope it will help you, and anyone else who reads it, become aware of the very nature of the healing process and the power you already possess to ignite it, embrace the process and finish the job.

Chapter One

_____

The First Healer I Ever Met

"What you are looking for is looking for you." Francis of Assisi

I have been practicing the healing arts since I was a child. Besides _playing doctor_ with the neighborhood kids, I remember putting my dolls through many different health challenges so I could _heal_ them. My medical kit came from the dime store and it had a lovely pink plastic stethoscope, a fake thermometer, imitation bandages, a harmless syringe, and one of those knee knocker gadgets real doctors use for checking reflexes. I poked and prodded my dolls, gave them injections, listened to their polyethylene hearts and bandaged their unbroken appendages. I even let one of my dolls _slip_ into the toilet one day so I could resuscitate her from the horrid accidental drowning . All of my dolls, regardless of the calamity, healed beautifully. But the joy of healing at home was nothing compared to what I learned when I was introduced to Violet Thornbush.

It was 1962 at the Shuskan Nursing Home in Bellingham, Washington. As a natural outcome of my healing successes with my dolls, when I was 13, along with my best friend Colleen, I became a Candy Striper (volunteer) after school at the local nursing home.

I plunged from play acting into real life with the speed of a whiplash. It was great, because, as a kid, I didn't really picture anyone as sick.

The patients just seemed old, grey haired, a bit infirm, missed the potty sometimes, and had strangers for roommates. It never occurred to me that this was a dreadful place, or anyone was at *death's doorstep* because I liked them, and I liked helping them do the things they couldn't do for themselves.

Most of the residents were grateful for the company and the little bit of assistance we gave them. We did simple things like change the linens and feed the patients who couldn't feed themselves. Sometimes we read letters from home, magazine articles, or chapters from their favorite books. Other times, we helped the nurses with patient related work and learned to assist with changing bandages and medicine distribution.

My friend Colleen spent extra time and took special care with a patient who kept asking her, *"I want some strawberries. Get me some strawberries."* Colleen, being the attentive Candy Striper, she was, one day brought her some fresh-picked strawberries from home. The patient promptly threw them against the wall.

Colleen, although flabbergasted by the action, carefully picked them up as the patient continued to ask for strawberries.

Perplexing as it was, some weeks later the intrepid Candy Striper finally figured out the patient was actually asking her to *wind her watch*. It was not about strawberries at all. Perhaps, in her own way, the elderly lady was just asking for more attention. Colleen was happy to wind her watch for her and give her what she needed.

Colleen was very helpful to all the residents, and to me. In my defense, I had never seen a men's bed urinal. Mr. Nordvert lived in a room by himself and he had this blue, conical container sitting on his tray. Thinking it was a vase, I generously offered to empty the *flower water* for him. I believe he smirked. He knew Colleen and had been a neighbor of hers before moving to the retirement facility. He told her of the incident. I'm sure they both had a good laugh. But Colleen, who was a foot taller than me, wrapped her kindly arm around my shoulder and led me to an area where we could speak in private.

She gently explained to me that *those blue cone-shaped containers* were not flower vases, but urinals for men who could not get out of bed to make it to the bathroom. "Oh," I shrieked, blushing like a schoolgirl in a horrific moment of discovery; which I was. Colleen made sure I was okay with the error and made me feel like I could face the world again, although I don't think I visited Mr. Nordvert's room again for at least 3 weeks.

But the best part of being a Candy Striper was the experience of Violet Thornbush. Violet was the nurse who ran the evening shift at the Shuksan Nursing Home. She showed up five days a week precisely at 4:30 pm.

There was never a need to check your watch, you knew exactly what time it was when Violet wheeled her turquoise truck into the reserved night staff parking space and came bursting through the *employees only* door.

It was like the mad rush of a flock of flapping seagulls. *Whoosh,* and there she was; singing loudly, smiling at everyone, cracking jokes, and making her way down the hall arm in arm with the elder folks who had camped out by the back door eagerly waiting for her. The day nurses hurried off, frowning when Violet arrived.

They couldn't miss the shift in the atmosphere, and they knew that the old folks couldn't wait for them to leave so the *Violet Hours* could begin. The day nurses left the building with scowls, dark expressions and a teensy bit of fear held tightly under their slickers, about what they might walk into in the morning or what there may be left to clean up after Violet's shift was over.

At 4:31 pm the world changed for the better at the Shuksan Nursing Home; it was like the Political Convention had just begun; complete with fancy party hats and squawking horns.

The patients couldn't wait for Violet to arrive, and neither could we. Violet didn't care if you were doing what you were *supposed to* be doing, all that she cared about was the spirit you brought to your job. The old men were hysterical. They started getting ready for Violet right after lunch trays were removed.

They preened, spritzed on the Old Spice, and perked up like proud squirrels with a new peanut when Violet time was near. To them, she was like Pamela Anderson on a USO tour. And Violet played fair; she charmed the ladies as well as the men with her wraparound smile and congeniality. She made everyone feel like dancing no matter who they were or what condition they were in.

But, in truth, I recall that the men may have perked up the most, because Violet did not believe in high necklines and made sure you saw as much of her tan as legally possible. Nurses' stockings were out of the question; it was bare legs all year around for this sun-loving beauty. Violet had no use for those crepe-soled white nurse's shoes; those lovely legs always terminated in a pair of something with heels that looked like they came from one of those glitzy shops on the Las Vegas strip. If it hadn't been for the facility's regulation white uniforms, I'm fairly sure Violet would have worn a leopard skin jumpsuit and a patent leather belt to work.

Her *whites* were always accented with some kind of a glamorous, sparkly neck scarf. In a different decade you might have thought of Violet as the pole-dancing night nurse. But here, she was simply Violet: the nurse with a flair for the spectacular.

The sun rarely shone in this part of the northwest but people at the Shuskan Nursing Home didn't care; Violet took its place. She was one happy-go-lucky barrel of fun and seemed always to be totally tickled with life. She specialized in medium length, blonde-streaked, salt and pepper hair that curled up naturally on the ends so it could keep to the beat of her bouncy walk. Her bottled Southern California tan stood out like a neon light in the middle of the cold, dreary, wet and rainy Pacific Northwest weather. A waft of floral air chased after Violet wherever she went. It suggested a generous application of the popular perfume *Tabu.*

The whole facility came suddenly alive, like a visit from the *Surprise Gardener*[2] to a dusty, barren, overgrown plot of land, when Violet clocked in. She was the breath of spring to folks in the winter of their lives. You never heard a complaint, a cranky remark, or a criticism during Violet's shift. The old folks were so busy waiting for her to come into their rooms on rounds; they didn't even think to complain.

A visit from Violet was ambrosia from the gods. She always had a smile, something to laugh about, authentic concern for their wellbeing and clever little stories. Although she had many tasks to accomplish on her shift, she gave time to everyone. She was a cloud of joy that morphed its way across every lonely bed and under each sullen door. Nobody minded getting their shots or taking their meds on Violet's shift. Everyone not just *felt* better but, when Violet was there, everyone *was* better. She was the first master healer I ever met.

My shift started at 3 pm, after school, and ended at 6pm. I only got to watch Violet at work for 90 minutes a day, two days a week, but the experience was enough to last a lifetime and to remember the feeling that I, and everyone else, had when she walked in the door.

One memory is particularly poignant. Resident Mary was much too thin, raggedly dressed, unkempt, with deep set, somewhat haunting eyes, and never was where she was supposed to be. She was the bane of the day nurses. Mary had some dementia and was always dragging a hand-made cloth dolly with her wherever she went. The dolly was about as raggedy-looking and threadbare as its owner.

---

[2] Television series where a team of gardeners mad a surprise visit to your unkempt backyard and turned it a monumental picture perfect scene.

Mary wandered; never outside, but always into places the day nurses didn't want her to be. They'd find her in the linen supply closet talking to her dolly, or under a kitchen table rocking her dolly, or locked in the nurses' bathroom singing to her dolly.

Sometimes Mary would visit other rooms, where often times she was neither invited nor welcome. There were certain times Mary was required to take specific medications and one was an injection. Mary hated the injections. Her skin was paper-thin and fragile, and she would scream when the day nurses would have to hold her down to give her the shots, if and when they could locate her.

I remember one nurse with a tightly wrapped bun and a guttural accent, who would search for Mary, find her, drag her like a naughty child into the dispensary, toss her dolly aside and tell her she couldn't have her doll back until she had taken all of her meds. The look of horror on Mary's face was permanently inscribed into my memory as she watched the nurse throw her precious doll on the floor.

Mary wailed and cried out with the anguish of a war-torn mother separated from her infant by menacing soldiers. Her calm returned only after she had taken her meds, received a band aid for the injection site and she was reunited with her dolly.

No such thing happened on Violet's shift. In fact, Mary often followed behind Violet on her rounds. I recall the chaos that ensued when Mary couldn't be located in time for the day nurses to administer her meds. Violet was instructed, by the exiting head day nurse, that Mary needed her full regimen.

"No problem," said Violet as she went about her business. Violet knew that Mary would eventually surface. Soon, Mary was following behind her and imitating her moves. Violet took Mary's hand and spoke directly to the dolly. She asked the dolly how she was today, she asked her how she was feeling, she asked if she was hungry and the dolly just shook her head, "No." Violet asked Mary if the dolly was telling the truth. Mary lightly shook her head, "No."

Violet asked Mary if she would help her get dolly something to eat. Mary agreed and off they went hand in hand. Violet sat with Mary while she *fed* the dolly and took a few bites herself to show dolly how it was done. When they came out of the dining room, Violet took Mary and the dolly to the dispensary where they gracefully took their meds and received their injections. Later, when Mary and the dolly tired of following Violet around, or forgot what they were doing, they went back to their room, cuddled up and fell asleep. Mary always slept soundly when Violet was on duty. I don't believe she slept at all when Violet had the night off.

Violet healed people. Aches and pains dissolved, depression and anxiety disappeared in her presence. Violet always seemed to know how to be and what to do. She wasn't somber or stressed in the face of illness, quite the contrary.

Violet faced confusion with confidence, disease with dignity and illness of all sorts with an expectancy of healing. Her positive attitude was contagious. Even in surroundings that some would consider the last frontier of hope, she summoned joy. Into an atmosphere of impending doom, Violet brought life.

Early on my understanding of the experience of healing was tied in the gift wrap of Violet's pure joy. I've never been able to separate the two. Whenever I have need for healing and I feel stymied or blocked, all I have to do is ask myself, "WWVD?" *What Would Violet Do*, and I have my answer straightaway.

Violet is inside of me. I was fortunate to catch a big dose of her and I am grateful for this active virus. Once I gather up the memory of Violet, her smile, her enthusiasm, the hugs she never denied anyone, her sequins and accoutrements, I know I'm just around the corner from total recovery. Violet's lessons live and breathe within me. Her joyous nature is how I experience healing. Some call that healing presence God, I call it my *Inner Violet* or "I.V." for short.

Joel Goldsmith wrote, "... *darkness isn't a thing, it doesn't exist, it is merely our experience of the absence of light, and it isn't present. Neither then is disease, poverty, malady, or lack because God did not create them, therefore they do not exist.*" If darkness is merely the absence of light, is illness, then, the absence of health? If they don't exist, why are they here?

They are here for two reasons. One is that many of us only truly appreciate something once we have lost it. By experiencing something off kilter and very human, perhaps even painful or uncomfortable, we often learn the lessons of our life. Those lessons are what bring us into our full human expression and the purpose of our journey this lifetime. (Nothing is wasted; it's all in how we choose to see it.)

The second reason is that we put our faith in the power of the visible world and not in the invisible Source of all life. Like the day nurses at the Shuksan Nursing Home, we are *just doing our jobs* but we are separating ourselves from the One Power that creates healing. We have to stop for a moment and remember our Inner Violet.

When Violet started her night duty, she arrived already aware that she was part of the whole. Violet, her job and those she ministered to were all the same thing. During her shift everybody mattered equally and was the same. She may have had the keys to the medicine cabinet, and she could come and go as she pleased, but in her mind she was on equal footing with the residents. That's why they loved her. She was all of them, and all for them. Violet was the healing Power in the place. The patients believed that and trusted that and were healed by that. When we forget about the One Source that healing comes from, we all need to call up our I.V. (Inner Violet) and allow ourselves to bask in it.

At some level we're all versions of Violet. Intrinsically we're all self-healers. Each of us may be an avenue for that all-smiling, all loving, empowering, gentle, giving, sharing, nurturing Presence. We are it and we may radiate it and, as we do, become more of the Power that we can unleash in our lives, in our minds, our bodies and in our worlds. It simply boils down to how we perceive and relate to our own *Inner Violet* and all of the residents in the cosmic nursing home called Life.

Remember Violet as we move through these pages. When you feel discouraged or overwhelmed (or not up to the task) just wait by the healing door and know that, at precisely the right moment, Violet, and all of her wisdom and healing wiles will pop through the door. She is right there; ready to walk arm in arm with you to guide you joyously into your wholeness.

Chapter Two

_____

Healing: Science or Art?

"The whole point of existence is not to fear God(s), or to worship God(s), but to become God(s)."   Marlene Morris

In our culture when we think about healing it would be normal to picture laboratories, x rays, pharmacies, operating rooms and hospitals. We are all familiar with the science of healing; from our favorite TV shows to mailboxes overflowing with offers to *heal something fast* all for $19.95, provided we make the call *right now*. But, when we get down to the nitty gritty of healing and consider the subject beyond the white coats and stethoscopes, what do we uncover? A big mystery!

Everyone alive has watched a wound heal and appreciated the body's ability to repair and restore a nasty gash in our flesh. But do we know how that healing happens or why it occurs? Can the healing process be explained by science or is it more like an art?

David Hawkins says in his book *Power Versus Force,* *"Medicine has forgotten that it was an art and that science was merely a tool of that art."* [3] When we allow the science to supplant the art, we approach healing backwards. Healing is then considered an accident, or a by-product of the tool, instead of the natural outcome of our artful efforts.

_____

[3] David Hawkins, *Power Versus Force*

Michelangelo's *David* is the masterpiece of an *artist*; the chisel and the marble are merely the tools used by the artist to achieve his full artistic expression. It is imperative that we think and act as an artist when we approach healing. Like Michelangelo, we need to understand that the art of healing comes from the wisdom that lives within our true self and not from mechanical, external tools.

The tools of science are meant to serve the healing arts, not the other way around. Often this hierarchy is difficult to discern because science has such a loud voice in our society. Science boasts of solutions and cures, but it is still called the *practice* of medicine because science is still *rehearsing*.
It requires courage to stand up against the powerful machine of science and say, *"You are here to serve me, not control me."* Science will boom back defensively and claim that all of its facts are verifiable. But science still cannot explain what actually occurs in healing; it remains a mystery. Science can describe the verifiable steps that occur in healing, but it can only *guess* at why.

Remember that science is a *Johnny-come-lately* to the party of existence. Before science there was art and the first artist was God. As Edward Young said, *"The course of Nature is the Art of God."* Let's approach healing then as the very Art of God.

In her book *Becoming God(s),* Marlene Morris uses the story of creation, broken down into the traditional seven days enumerated in the Bible, to illustrate the steps of cosmic and personal creation. First there was awareness and then came light. Then when there was light there came firmament, and the waters, and the land, then the grasses, the fruit trees and the creatures of the land and air and water and finally, humanity.

Each day God called what It had made *"Good"* and then, on the 7th day, God rested and allowed the creation to continue, to pick up the process and to make more of the same. The book details our path of individual creation as we move through seven stages from believing we are *"mere mortals"* into our true state of Godliness.

We were made in the image and likeness of God and we are tasked with remembering the journey of creation back to the light, the wholeness, from whence we came. The book describes the creative process in terms we can understand, step by step. As we take those steps, we find that we arrive at our original, natural state.

The art of creation is akin to the art of healing. Both are processes of indeterminable length; they can happen in an instant or over the span of a lifetime. (Seven days could have been billions of years, or it could have been overnight. We don't know.)

Both develop according to intention. Ultimately the first act of creation made something out of nothing; the act of healing is a return to the purest state, unmaking what has shown up in the body as imbalance or what we call illness. For healing to be achieved, as we move through the steps, we must do what God did and identify each new unfolding layer as *Good*. We must realize that each step we take towards our return to wholeness is praiseworthy; each step is as important and as necessary as each of the six days of creation, and just as remarkable.

At the core of healing is the act of co-creating our physical universe, with God, one day at a time. We don't have to start all of creation from scratch; God already accomplished that, we only have to remember the pure essence of who we are, do what is before us to do, and allow Grace to fill in the rest. The saying *"by the Grace of God"* is more meaningful than ever in healing, because this Divine grace is not a man-made science, it is an art. We can change the phrase and make even a more powerful statement by altering one word, "by the Grace *in* God."

The implication is crystal clear. Grace in God is inclusive of everyone. We operate by the Grace in God and *as* the Grace in God. Grace is just another term for the quintessence of God. Grace is not bequeathed; it is discovered and released.

Grace springs forth as a gift when you focus on the inner work of your soul. Every day you can seize the opportunity to go deeper inside, to pray, to connect with your spiritual self and to know God.

This is not an impossible task; it simply requires time, attention and belief. Make the time and you will create the atmosphere for Grace. Once you allocate the time to listen to your inner voice and to connect with Spirit, the condition will shift, it has to.

Change comes, and Grace is the power behind *how* the change will manifest. You are the healing artist, how will you choose to use the spiritual tool of grace? The path of healing is the same path as that of the artist. The form of the sculpture rises out of the marble; the form of the healing rises out of the inner healer; the artist is a mere tool for its revelation. What will *your* masterpiece be?

Grace can show up anywhere, because it *is* everywhere. Whether or not we tap into it and allow it to operate through us, is up to us. Carolyn Myss says, *"Grace emerges out of your own inner work and the healing of dark passions. It comes through prayer and through discovering that you thrive more on truth than on fear."*[4] Myss further notes that Teresa of Avila spoke of Grace as something that we no longer have to dig for because, as we develop a rich interior life, Grace is endlessly supplied.

If we cannot mine for Grace or dig for it, how do we find it? Where is it and how can we get some? When we believe that Grace is supplied in unlimited quantity, we have confidence that conditions can transform, and we can heal.

---

[4] Carolyn Myss, *Defying Gravity*

The mind and the body alone cannot *cure* illness; but with Divine Power as God, Spirit or Grace, health can be restored resulting in harmony and balance. What is essential is the cultivation of your receptive soil, so that when Grace appears, you are open to accept it, like the garden is for the seed.

At birth we seem helpless and dependent, we must look to someone else for our needs. We confuse our biological or substitute parents for our real Source. We grow up believing things outside of us make us who we truly are. Our identity is mirrored by our environment. Sometimes we believe in the ways of man instead of the steps to God. We forget that we are connected to, and filled with, the Source of our Creation.

The Light of the Creator dims in comparison to the neon lights of the world. And then one day we feel lonely, empty. We begin to search for meaning. We want to become something or someone. We buy a book, we take a class, we travel to a distant land looking for a way and a means to fill the gap. The real secret that we eventually uncover is that we don't really ever need to *become* anything.

Our lives are a series of revelations from the inside out. Some of us pay attention to the lessons of our lives; others miss the point entirely. In her book, Dr. Morris uses the word *becoming* as both a noun and a verb. In actuality, we spend our lives living experiences that are meant to reawaken the Truth of whom and what we are, and what we are capable of becoming.

The *science* behind *becoming* is well documented in the theory of evolution. Life begins as one cell and through a series of duplications, evolves into a living, breathing collection of cells.

Through multiplication and growth, we become physical humans, animals, and creatures of all shapes and sizes. The art of becoming *is* the art of healing in that healing is a process of revealing the Truth already present.

To *become* is to reveal inner Truth; to heal is to unmask the illness - and reveal wholeness. Healing, however, is an individual art because, unlike evolution, the process unfolds differently for each person. What may heal one person may not heal another.

The healing artist uses intuition, instinct, and an inner voice to explore the ramifications of healing and to guide the process with care and compassion; appreciating not only that which is being healed, but the very process of healing itself. Healing is Divine work by nature and therefore cannot be accessed by human means alone. True healing comes from the spiritual realms where Grace resides. The gift of Grace is waiting for you to accept it.

Mastering the art of healing is to gently peel away the layers that suppress the emergence of the inner healer. As we lift the veils that block our connection to the Divine, we step deeper into the realm of true healing. And we want desperately to do that don't we? We want a deeper connection, a vivid experience of the healer within. We want to taste the miraculous and drink from the cup of divine ambrosia to lift our burdens and lighten our hearts where pains disappear and struggles dissolve in an instant and we would live in a constant state of Grace. Isn't that our dream?

No matter what your present condition is as you turn these pages, the above description is not as farfetched as you may feel it to be. *Supreme Healing* teaches you how to cultivate your personal resources for creating the identical state. One of the tools through which you can do that is *Becoming God(s)*.

Becoming God(s) is a magnificent guide to the art of healing. It is the conscious voyage of returning home. When we fully return to our original Essence, we heal from anything that is not made of Pure Spirit. When we *become* what we actually are but have forgotten in the course of our lives, we live immersed in grace. When we *become*, we *heal*.

Let us *fortify* our soil, *become* Gods, *accept* Grace, and *heal* our lives, beginning in our minds.

Chapter Three

_____

The Healing Mindset

"Every situation properly perceived, becomes an opportunity to heal." A Course in Miracles

Before we begin to investigate the process of healing, it may be helpful for us to take a chapter to discuss the properties of healing. I'd like to introduce this section with thoughts from Dr. Serge King's book, _Kahuna Healing_. The word kahuna means _healer_ in Hawaiian. Dr. King is a renowned Kahuna: a shaman, teacher and healer. He was trained by shamanic healers in Hawaii and around the globe. He was one of my teachers and I value the work he proliferates in the world. The Kahuna practice and philosophy begins with the interior beliefs and mental atmosphere of a person and works its way out, much like Chinese medicine.

Dr. King writes, "_Hawaiian Kahuna healing involves the whole person - the Higher Self, the conscious mind, the subconscious and the body - and the person's environment. Since its purpose is to bring about a healing and not prove a particular method, it is geared to individual needs. The same Kahuna (healer) might use different methods to treat two people with identical symptoms because their beliefs might be quite different. And beliefs, according to Huna, are at the root of all illness._"

When we give this statement the weight it deserves, an entire universe of possibility opens up. We link the Body, Mind and Heart in an inseparable triangle of activity.

These are not random parts of the human being, but integrated, interwoven, interlocked sections that function as a complimentary and interdependent system. Plato said, *"The part can never be well unless the whole is well."* This is also the core of the Kahuna belief system.

Dr. King continues to explain that, *"The Kahunas have an unorthodox view of the effects of medicine based on their idea that illness is not caused by bacteria, viruses or carcinogenic agents, but by tension resulting from conflicts of thought and emotional energy."*

"A conflict of thought and emotional energy." What implications might that have on the healing process? What if disease was caused not by the germs we encounter, but by what we are thinking, and how we are managing the stresses and conflicts in our lives? What if our body, by becoming ill, is trying to send us a signal that we need a better balance of body, mind and heart? The approach for healing, as well as continued well-being, catapults us into an entirely new area of self-care and a process of internal healing that trumps external methods.

Just think of what might become of our lives if suddenly we turned inside ourselves for solutions and were no longer dependent on the external ones?
Can you imagine how the world would be if we began with the mind and the heart and worked our way to the outside body?

What might happen in your life if you turned within to seek healing solutions and thereby you took full control of your emotions, feelings and actions, resulting in the prevention of many stressful situations that weaken your constitution and leave you susceptible to illness?

This would lead you into a new focus on wellness where you are not just cognizant of, but responsible for, your own health and healing. Your mind would be strengthened, your choices inner- based and your actions congruent with your thoughts. You could live in harmony and balance; healthy from the inside out. What a concept!

Let us look deeper into Dr. King's writings. *"The Kahunas do not claim that germs and microbes do not exist, but that they are catalysts and by-products of disease and not its cause. If there were no fear or undue tension in people, there would be no disease regardless of the presence of bacteria or viruses associated with the illness."*[5]

Is that statement a stretch to believe? If it is, then please stretch. Having no contact that we know of with a Kahuna, Louis Pasteur agreed.

He wrote, *"The germ is nothing; the soil is everything."* Meaning that some people become infected when exposed to a virus or bacteria and others do not. The soil is what matters the most not the germ.

"The Kahunas teach that belief complexes[6] act as guidance systems for the flow of the life force, Mana. Where there is conflict, the flow is distorted and this distortion may lead to acute or chronic tension on a muscular, organ or cellular level.

---

[5] Serge King, *Kahuna Healing*

[6] Meaning: structures of beliefs or patterns.

Such tension can lead to pain and illness. That is why the Kahunas believe the source of all illness can be found in conflicting ideas. Hawaiian for illness is Ma'i meaning a 'state of tension or restriction....the Kahuna word for healing is ola, best translated as 'enlightenment' (o - to enter; la - light)."[7]

Healing is in fact enlightenment, *entering the light.* This light is not something we can touch or feel, but we may step into it, and be surrounded and illuminated by it. We become united with it. It speaks silently yet produces profound results because we are ever changed by our integration with it. If we take our enlightenment seriously, healing becomes an easy result from this junction.

Kahunas believe that ideas or thoughts do not become materially effective unless they become part of your mind on all levels: conscious and subconscious.

"Knowledge which remains intellectual is nothing more than opinion."[8] And we all know opinion has no effect for change on the individual or the world. Healing, in the Kahuna world, *"comes as a natural result of allowing the God energy to flow through oneself in the original pattern of the spiritual body. Illness and distortion of any kind result when that flow is interrupted."* [9] When we are centered in the conviction that Spirit is All that exists, is the only Power, the Complete Knowledge and All Perfection, then how can we hold, at the same time, ~~that disease and illness are~~ real?

[7] Serge King, *Kahuna Healing*

[8] Ibid

[9] Serge King, *Kahuna Healing*

The Kahunas certainly believe it isn't. In essence when we are convinced that Spirit is the All, is the only real Power, then it becomes impossible to believe that disease and illness are more than temporary situations. When we accept the idea emotionally as well as intellectually, we open unprecedented avenues for healing.

The Kahunas look to the mind as the first source of imbalance. They encourage becoming aware of one's thoughts and know that if healing is to occur it will only come about when a pattern of thinking is shifted into a new pattern that opens the flow of God (mana) within.

To encourage that shift in consciousness one of the ways Kahunas begin the healing process is to give the patient *mana-charged* water to drink. *Mana* is the Hawaiian word for Divine power. Kahunas believe in the *secret life of water*. They believe the molecules in water accept the energy infused into it by focused concentration emanating from the mind and the heart of the healer.

The water is infused with the spirit of Aloha (love) and Divine power (mana). The Kahunas suffuse plain water with their thoughts and the breath of life, while focusing intently on a healing image. The water is given to the patient to drink so that it may trigger a shift in his or her belief and in doing so release the flow of God, Mana, within them. The Kahunas believe that *"true healing is a shifting of beliefs and when that takes place the cure is permanent."*[10]

---

[10] Ibid

"If treatment fails it only means that there has not been a deep enough thought or change in the person's mind. Perhaps the resistance is that the benefit of the cure is far more painful (or perceived as such) than living with the current illness." [11]

What is more important to you than allowing the healing to occur? What might you be holding onto that is more important than your healing; what is it that might be blocking the Spirit of God flowing through you at the highest level? If healing is dependent upon your consciousness and your openness to the flow of the Divine Power within, what is it that you must be conscious of? Let us consider the eight beliefs that comprise your healing mindset. The understanding of these statements will carry you into the next three phases of healing.

It will serve you well to take the time to commit these to memory and use them as the infrastructure for your healing journey. They have been inspired by some of Dr. King's teachings, enlightened by the Kahuna traditions, The Science of Mind, and furthered developed by my own work.

The Beliefs of the Healing Mind Set are:

1) Healing is Truth revealing itself.
2) Healing is what you believe it is.
3) There are no limits to what can be healed.
4) Healing goes where Spirit flows.
5) At the center of healing is love.
6) All healing comes from within.

---

[11] Ibid

7) ASK, (Assume Spirit's Knowledge) and it shall be given to you.
8) Healing begins when you say it does.

As we explore what each of these statements means let us see how they can open us to a healing consciousness that reaches far beyond what we have believed or thought before.

1) Healing is Truth revealing itself.

Healing is the act of Divine Wholeness revealing Itself within us. Healing is becoming aware of, and releasing, that which we already possess. Think about it, if God is within then we already have everything we need and all that is required for healing is the release of that inner Power. But when we are not cognizant of this Power, or when we have shut down to it, invaders fill the empty space. Instead of releasing the power within we compress it, thus leaving us vulnerable to unwelcome visitors.

Invaders come in many forms such as illness, unhappiness, poverty, fear, and despair. We must become aware that these are not part of our intrinsic wholeness, but rather are the effect of a detour in consciousness.

About his own healing, David R. Hawkins writes, *"It appeared that physical illness was really the result of negative belief systems and that the body could actually literally change as a result of the shift of a belief pattern. One is really subject to what is held in mind."* [12]

---

[12] David R. Hawkins, *The Eye of the I*

The effects of the invaders are felt at the physical level, but the source for healing is on the God level. Healing is the natural byproduct of our conscious choice to allow God to express as health through our minds, hearts and bodies.

For the Divine within this is not work; it is effortless; it is natural. The only work involved in healing is to make room for the Power to manifest; to clear out the clutter. We may be required to change our old beliefs and replace them with empowering thoughts once we decide this is the place we want to live. A good start it to change your mental address to: *#1 God Street* and start acting as though you are a permanent resident.

Ultimately when we believe that God is All there is and that the healing Presence lives inside of us, we have nothing left to do but connect to that Divine Presence and allow It to reveal the true wholeness of our being. When we consciously set our illness beliefs aside and let the Inner God shine forth, wholeness is automatically revealed.

Exercise

Close your eyes and visualize the TV set from "To Tell The Truth". (For those of you who need a refresher, the show featured a celebrity panel on the left, a host on the right, and in the middle three people who claimed to be *the guest* were seated, and only one swore to *tell the truth*.

The host read a mini biography of the guest in the first person. (Sample) *"I, Orville Redenbacher, was born in **Brazil, Indiana**, and grew up on my family's farm where I sometimes sold **popcorn** from a roadside stand. I joined **4-H**, and developed an **obsession** for discovering the perfect **popping corn**. I attended **Purdue University** and graduated with a degree in **agronomy** in 1928. My popcorn is the #1 selling brand in America."*

Each of the three imposters on the center dais was given an allotted time to answer questions from the celebrity panel. At the end of the questioning each of the panelists voted on whom they thought was the real Orville Redenbacher. Once the votes were cast, the host asked, *"Will the real Orville Redenbacher please stand up?"*

The real guest stood, and the two impostors then revealed their real names and their actual occupations. Prize money was awarded to the challengers based on the number of *incorrect* votes they drew.)

With your eyes closed ask the following questions:

> 1. If I were to appear as a guest on this game show (who is sworn to tell the truth) what would I tell about my belief in healing?
> 2. Would I be willing to *speak* my Truth?
> 3. Could I defend that the Truth within me as the Power and Presence of Spirit?
> 4. Do I believe I am who I say I am?
> 5. Do I need more convincing about the healing within me?
> 6. How would the panel vote based on my answers?

Your answers should reveal to you the level of confidence you have about the nature of healing. If they are not what you want them to be, do not give up, keep reading. There is simply more to learn.

2) Healing is what you believe it is.

What is healing for you? Is it the alleviation of pain, removal of symptoms, complete freedom from any effect of disease or restriction? What do you expect healing to accomplish? Only you can define what your healing looks like, feels like and is.

Your *belief* that you have the power within you to manifest healing will attract whatever resources you may need. But understand that material resources (anything from band aids to prescription medicine) do not do the healing.

The healing comes from *within you*. If you have been raised to believe that some authority outside of you does the healing, then you have work to do. The only *authority* you need in order to heal is the Authority of Spirit that you already possess. It came with your original packaging and instructions.

But like many instructions we don't always read them prior to assembly and therein lies the reason why we end up with a part or two missing. You have no need to worry. The instructions for healing are available all the time, everywhere, to anyone. It is important that you take time to understand and acknowledge your beliefs as they are now because what you believe leads directly to the environment of healing. Your beliefs create your mental soil. Let's discover what you believe healing is.

Exercise

Please complete the following sentences:

The definition of healing is:
_____

My source of healing is:
_____

I have experienced healing:
_____

To heal I have to:
_____

I need to heal.
_____

I cannot heal without:
_____

My healing looks like
_____

I will heal when
_____

My definition of healing is:
_____
_____
_____

Be very honest with your answers and then take a look at them in light of the following:

Healing is an act of Grace and Divine Wholeness revealing itself within us.

Allow a few moments to integrate the power of this statement. This is the basic truth you need to accept for healing to occur. If you want to alter your belief(s) at any time to enhance the properties of your mental soil, you'll have the opportunity in Chapter Six. For now, make notes of what you want to change.

3) There are no limits to what can be healed.

This is a simple equation: God is Whole; the Power of God is unlimited in the Universe, in us, in everything; therefore, everything and anything can be healed. What was created can always be recreated and healed.

Healing is ultimately the return to original wholeness. Healing simply reinstates the spiritual status quo, which is entire and complete Perfection.

The only limitation to healing is what the human mind determines it is.

If you think a condition or a situation cannot be healed; it won't be. If you believe in the endless possibility of creation and recreation you will become visibly aware of it in action. You know this principle is true in everyday life.

Once you buy a particular brand of car you begin to notice more of them as you drive around. This is also true of your beliefs.

Once you focus on a specific belief, it begins to increase in your awareness, and you send off signals that attract more of the same into your field of attention and consciousness. Focus attention on one thing in your life and observe closely as more of it appears.

Healing is a personal matter. It summons the private sage in a fervent call to belief and action. Your job is to elevate your beliefs to lofty heights and keep them there.

If someone in your world reels off discouraging statistics or uses words like *terminal, deadly, fatal, incurable,* or *chronic,* tune them out. They are not functioning on your new wavelength. Ask them to support you and your concept of *unlimited potential.*

If they don't, then take a vacation from them, change the channel, and allow in only the thoughts and ideas which support your belief in the endless and unlimited power of recreation, restoration, revitalization, recovery and renewal.

Exercise:

Imagine: *It is your birthday. You are dressed in the most splendid array of garments you can imagine. You are surrounded by beings of light. Sounds of harmonious singing fills the air. You are warm, safe, comfortable, and at peace. Joy is welling up inside of you and you are the focus of all attention in the room. Notice a table at the end of the room.*

On it is a fountain with cascading waters which flow up from inside and down along the sides. One of the light beings picks up the fountain and brings it to you. This being is accompanied by others, all happy to be part of the presentation. This fountain is light as a feather, yet it miraculously pumps the sparkling water in and out, up and down in a seemingly endless supply. You hold it on your lap, it is weightless, there are no visible cords and yet it continues to flow. You dance around the room with it. You toss it back and forth among the light beings and it continues to flow. It is miraculous; it never stops and there are no parts to break or batteries to change. It is a wonder. The light beings tell you that the fountain represents the healing power of Spirit which is in you and is constantly supplying you with the unlimited flow of life and Divine Love. It is eternal and can never be stopped. The power accompanies you wherever you go giving you an endless supply of itself. It is yours to keep; this fountain and the power it represents.   May it be your constant reminder that you have the power within you to heal anything anytime.

Return to this simple vision anytime you have a limiting thought or have started to believe in someone else's opinion about healing that is not in tune with your belief that the possibilities for healing are limitless.

4) Healing goes where Spirit flows.

Healing power is the presence of God in Action. If we dam a river, the water goes where we direct it. The same is true for *Mana*, Divine Power. If limiting beliefs and emotions are blocking the flow of our healing supply, or unconsciously re-routing it, we need to clear the path and consciously allow the original flow to resume.

Healing flows where Spirit is free to express. Our mental fences are the only structures that keep it corralled. Unlock the dam and Spiritual Power abounds." *Through choices human consciousness can influence outcomes, but the power of creation is the province of God."*[13]

Exercise:

Close your eyes and focus on your breath. Set your intention to relax. Inhale five times   until you feel your body relax. (Inhale for 5 seconds and exhale for 5 seconds) Imagine that you contain the breath of God. When you have relaxed, turn your attention to your knees. Breathe into your knees for three long, sustained breaths.(Pause) Next, turn your attention to your hands. Breathe into your hands for three long, sustained breaths. (Pause) Now, turn your attention to the back of your neck muscles and breathe into them for three long sustained breaths. (Pause) Now, turn your attention to your stomach. Take three long sustained breaths and breathe into it. (Pause) Lastly, take three longs breaths as you focus on your cheek muscles on your face. Breathe into that area and pause.

The parts of your body that you focused on should be feeling more relaxed and at ease than the rest of your body. Where you focused concentrated breathing and attention should have given you release and relaxation.

---

[13] David R. Hawkins, *The Eye of the I*

As you focus your attention onto a body part, a belief, a desire or a mental picture, it will receive that attention and the Life energy of Spirit will flow to it. You create a current of healing when you fix your attention on a person, place, part or thing. Centered concentration can bring about a shift in a condition. Direct your spiritual energy where you want it, and it will comply.

5) At the center of healing is love.

God, by definition, is the essence of Love. We participate in that Divine Loving Presence in the *feelings* of love that we experience. Along with our experience of love, and the associated feelings, is the wholeness that the fullness of the expression of Love provides. It is in the atmosphere of Love that healing occurs. *"Merely thinking thoughts of appreciation won't make the change...The Law of Love does not operate on thoughts of love. It only operates on feelings of love."*[14] You've got to feel it to achieve it.

To fully experience, we must create a neutral field wherein nothing blocks our acceptance of Love expressing Itself. We must rid our minds of negative thoughts like resentment, fear, hatred, and envy, in order to provide a receptive atmosphere wherein Love can reside. There is human work to do, but the rewards are spiritual, and they are key to unlocking the healing process.

Being in the Presence of someone filled with Love is a remarkable experience. Suddenly our cracks are filled in and we no longer feel the drafts of loneliness and separation.

---

[14] David MacArthur & Bruce MacArthur, *The Intelligent Heart*

We are engulfed by this warm and welcoming ambiance and our hearts are lifted in joy. There is no reason we can't feel this way all the time.

The Hawaiians call it the Spirit of Aloha. *"Love is a way of acting toward and with others, and a way of feeling about yourself and others. The way of acting is always a healing one, encouraging the object of love to thrive and grow; the way of feeling is always a happy and joyful one. You could say then that to love is to heal, and to heal is to love."*[15]

To love, then, becomes a choice. When you make the choice in your mind to open your heart, you release the love outward.

Exercise:

Close your eyes and picture the most loving experience you have ever had. Recall everything you can about the situation; the time frame, the weather, the location, the people. When you have that picture in your mind, sit with it for a moment, filling in all of the mental details you can. (Give it about 30 seconds) When you have the picture vivid in your mind, turn your focus to your heart. Notice how it feels, notice how the feeling spreads throughout your body. Make note of any other sensations you feel. (Give this about 30 seconds)

When you have established your recognition of the feelings of love coming from your heart, change your mental picture to a recent mildly unpleasant experience you have had.

---

[15] Serge King, *Kahuna Healing*

Perhaps an occasion that was embarrassing, painful or awkward for you. Now, quickly bring your heart energy up into your mind. Take all the feelings of love and happiness and raise them up into your mental region.

Let the love fill your memory. Notice anything that changed in your experience of the negative memory. Notice what shifted when you brought love into the picture. Take a moment to move around in your memory and note any differences in the situation. (Give it about 30 seconds)

When you have completed this exercise, the results should leave you feeling better about the unpleasant situation. The loving feelings you brought to the memory altered and neutralized it.

This exercise can be used to preview activities in our lives and bring love to an uncomfortable or feared situation. It can be used as a tool to create the approach we wish to take and enjoy the result we want to have.

Picture in your mind any situation you are in, or about to be in, or were in; fire up the feeling of love in your heart and bring that love directly up into your mental picture. You can change your moment, your day and your future by depositing love precisely where you want it. You will make your decisions and choices from this heart set rather than from any other place. "We can achieve different effects and experiences by shifting our focus from one dimension or level to another."[16]

6) All healing comes from within.

---

[16] Serge King, *Kahuna Healing*

If you still hang on to the belief that healing will come as a result of something outside yourself, healing will not come. Healing is the release of *your* inherent spiritual power. It is your birthright. You are a living, breathing, member of the Kingdom of God and it is that very essence you hold within yourself that is unlimited and has but one requirement: release. *Believe* that you hold the power within and then seek ways to consciously release and experience it.

Supreme Healing begins with your *recognition* of the living Spirit within, allowing the revelation of that to be your Truth, combined with your unfailing belief that your actual healing comes solely from the Spirit within and nowhere else.

When you honestly feel that you have given up indulgence in any feelings of anger, hate, jealousy, resentment, malice or other negative emotions, and you are completely in an atmosphere and state of being that is receptive to spiritual healing, then and only then, when your consciousness is open to and participating in the internal flow of Spirit, will you heal.

Giving up negative feelings does not require arduous quantities of effort. You can shift your perspective and focus on Love as the Source of your healing and wholeness as simply as putting on a pair of reading glasses. The secret of healing lies in the fine print, and you may just need to magnify your thoughts about healing, wholeness and Spirit in order to participate in the terms required for healing. The answer comes when you recognize that you are both the healer and the healed.

"The healing ability is, in fact, the evidence that we are spiritual beings." [17] Wholeness is the spiritual heritage of our cells. You can block it by harboring negative or limiting thoughts, but you cannot escape it. Choose to be on the accepting side. Allow your wholeness to reveal itself inside of you and demonstrate fully at the level of *Supreme Healing.*

Exercise

Believe with me, and join me in knowing: (most powerful when read aloud)

Spirit is not separate from me; it shares my shoes. We walk together as One and we are called by the same name. As much as God is in me; I am in God, also. When I allow the Presence, that active Spirit, to engage in all of my activities, to attend all functions, to permeate all thoughts and to generate all action, there is no separate me, there is us, thinking, acting, doing and believing as One. I become the perfect party of One.

Continue to repeat the statement out loud until you *believe* it!

7) *ASK*, (Assume Spirit's Knowledge) and it shall be given to you.

---

[17] Eric Mein, M.D. *Keys to Health*

When you **ASK** (see Chapter Four) you will find that everything is supplied to you. When you accept that the Life within you is the Life of Spirit, then you can easily download anything from the unlimited body of healing knowledge that Spirit has. You have been afforded a lifetime of unlimited access to all of the power and the knowledge in the Universe. Open any file, anytime and it's yours to absorb and explore.

When you **A**ssume **S**pirit's **K**nowledge you are instituting a positive mental and spiritual action; one wherein you connect the dots between your power and the Power of God.

If God is all there is, and God is All Knowledge, it follows that if God is in you all the time, then all of God's knowledge is there, too. You have every right to **A**ssume **S**pirit's **K**nowledge as your own. It's your birthright. The act of *asking* takes on a different perspective when it originates from that position of spiritual entitlement. This is the perfect example of entitlement and assumption. Assume you have the Knowledge so it can come *through* you.

Do not confuse the issue: this *asking* is not begging or beseeching an outside deity to *fix* your life; it is assuming your spiritual entitlement for all of the right reasons. Having a driver's license is a privilege; knowing and believing that you share in Divine Knowledge is your right.

Exercise:

> *Answer True or False to the following questions:*

Knowledge is something that belongs to Spirit and not to me.

If I ask Spirit nicely, I might be given the answer.

All answers to the great questions are locked up.

Spirit has the secret key.

If I pray hard enough Spirit will rescue me.

I have to study harder in order to get the answers to my healing.

I may have to wait for the answers until Spirit is ready to give them to me.

I may not be important enough for Spirit to help me.

Other people may be more deserving the I am.

I depend on Spirit to fix things in my life; even if I broke them, Spirit has to fix them.

There is always a long line waiting for Spirit.

All of the answers are *false*. If you answered *true* to any one of them, you need a quick review. Please read this chapter from the beginning and take the test again!

8) Healing begins when you say it does.

---

[18] Serge King, *Kahuna Healing*

"The Kahunas teach that the present is the fruit of the past, and the seed of the future... The future grows out of what is happening now."[18] If you carefully examine the present, you can predict your future.

If you believe in the power of the present, you can dissect what is going on right now in your mind, body and heart, and determine your future. Whatever you are thinking and doing right now determines the outcome tomorrow.

Think about that statement and give some additional consideration as to what you are thinking in this moment, right now. Quickly inventory your present thoughts. What is in your mind on the following subjects: health; well-being; happiness; contentment; abundance; self-approval? Check in with yourself to measure where your thoughts right now. What do they tell you?

In healing there is no past, there is only the present. What has or has not been done, or said, or healed, is history. When you open yourself to experience the Power, the Presence acts for you in that moment. *Now* is the only moment you have. This is the instant of connection to the Power of God. Eckhart Tolle says,

"The quality of your consciousness at this moment is what shapes the future — which, of course, can only be experienced as the Now"[19]

The past is gone; the future is a blank canvas to be painted on by a creative thought in Mind. *Now*, this moment, is the only true reality you have.

---

[19] Eckhart Tolle, *The Power of Now*

A major key to healing is the recognition that you can do nothing with the past. It is over, it is gone, it is done. The opportunity you have at hand is to alter the future in this very instant. When you consciously seize that opportunity in this moment you begin the healing process *instantaneously*.

This is not something you do in your intellect alone; you must feel it, taste, it and embody the moment of now in the depths of your soul in order for the Power to flow and release.

Your healing begins at the exact moment you claim your inner Power and purposefully unleash the flow of Spirit. Your human mind controls the timing and the release button. When you say, "*Now is the time*," the process begins. It is effective immediately.

Chapter Four

_____

Conviction: The First Act in Healing

"There are only two ways to live your life. One is as though nothing is a miracle. The other as though everything is a miracle." Albert Einstein

Just as there are generally three acts in a play, there are also three steps, or *acts* to healing. In a play the separate acts are used to define a change of location or time; they are also orchestrated for the sake of dramatic impact, juxtaposition and coherent storytelling. The acts in a play build upon each other to tell the complete story as the playwright designed. Similarly, one of the central characteristics in the healing process is that the steps also lead one to the other and evolve out of one another.

As artists of our own well-being, let us examine the first quality, or *act* in our healing play: Conviction. To arrive at Conviction, we begin as all good authors do; we establish the environment. In healing we must set up the environment of our belief system, define where it originates, what truths it encompasses and how our beliefs and truths define the world we inhabit. In terms of playwriting, this is the platform for the author to establish and articulate the world in which the story abides.

Once we have comprehended the qualities and the scope of this created *world*, then the action and the dialog can commence. In a play we are made aware of the time, the location and, if well written, the mindset of the era exemplified by how the characters think and behave. From this point on, the scenes mentally and emotionally carry us forward across the pinnacles and crevices of the plot. It is in the combination of the characters, their virtues and flaws, compounded with the interaction of other characters and situations, and through the evolvement of the play that we learn the truths (lessons) the writer wishes to convey. Healing is similar.

Consider a play about Elizabeth I. The writer sets up the location so we understand clearly that the era is 16th century England. The writer enriches this setting by way of costumes, locations, sets and makeup. We are introduced to the situation either via a narrative or by way of information that the characters convey in their dialog and demeanor.

Queen Elizabeth enters the throne room, people curtsy; we understand who is who and we witness the customs of the realm. The manner and tone in which the characters speak to each other establishes status, class and position. The scene is set, if you will, for the era, the hierarchy of power, and placement of the various characters within the constructed scene.

The problems that the characters must deal with or are asked to solve over the course of the play, are the keys to the evolution of their characters and the forward movement of the plot.

The manner in which they handle the challenges gives us further insight into their strengths and weaknesses as we follow the passages they are asked to endure throughout the course of the play. By their choices and behavior, they will succeed or fail; they will end up victorious, enslaved or dead.

As in playwriting, the same three act process is true for healing. The first act establishes the environment, the thoughts, beliefs, characters and the action. The second act defines the challenges, presents more tests, furthers the action and highlights the questions and unresolved issues in the minds of the audience. The third act answers the questions, resolves those issues and arrives at a conclusion, lesson or moral. The finale follows and is accompanied by deafening applause, thereby affirming artistic success, that the message was received.

Now let us apply this same creative process to our healing. The first act is Conviction. In the very first stage of our healing we must establish the Conviction that there is a Power greater than the thing which we wish to heal; that this Power is all there is; we set the parameters of the scene for our mind.

There is nothing outside of Supreme Energy; It is in and through everyone and everything. It is, for the purpose of healing especially, within us. Just as with the premise of a play, we may need further convincing of that principle. A good playwright describes the world in which the characters live, their passions, their foibles, their attitudes, perhaps even their past, in order to make us feel like we are part of their world; suspended with them in time and space.

So too, in establishing Conviction we must learn to place all of our faith and belief in the immediate Presence of the One and the Only. If we believe that Spirit has a part time job, or makes exceptions, or perhaps does not always work the way we want it to work, then we will not be able to successfully move onto the next step. The steps of healing progress one to the other, and without the primary foundation of Conviction, the second and third stages will not function effectively for us.

We must craft the foundation of our play and establish a premise we believe in before we can go onto compose the dialog and cast our spiritual healing play. We must, at the core of our essence, create the unflappable belief that The Power of God is all that exists in our Universe.

In order to create that belief and build up our Conviction of this irrefutable Truth, we need to cultivate an inner assurance that Spirit is the Absolute Truth and there is nothing else other than God at the Source and Center of all existence.
We must not just speak the words, as a character might in a play, but we must *believe* them with all our heart. In the theater of our mind, our world and all of our actions must revolve around this belief.

Conviction, in this case, is the purest, solitary essence of the belief that there is only One Source of Life, One Center of Power, One Fountain of Supply and that the Living Source of our healing is God.

When the bills are due, when a cherished friend or relative dies, when the wolf is banging on the door, when we are holding the winning ticket to a multi-million dollar lotto jackpot, when we are dancing up a storm, or celebrating our wildest dream come true; whatever we are doing and wherever we are at all times we must maintain the unshakeable, inherent knowledge that *this situation* is God working through us and in our lives.

This active God is constantly working through us and is completely Present, 100%, all of the time. No matter what is going on, or who is doing what to whom, our Faith must remain unflappable. Go there; stay there.

If we were able, during our darkest times and during the times of our greatest joys, to believe fully that Spirit is working through us and for us at all times, we would not have to rely on Tums or Rolaids to relieve our acid producing, limited, worry-wart, left brained, controlling, angst-ridden lives. Instead, we would just be able to *ride out* the fun, and not-so-fun times, alike and understand fully that we are Godlings having a poignant and agreeable human experience, regardless of the type of activity that is going on. Or, more aptly, according to the Harold Arlen song: *"Come Rain or Come Shine."*

Conviction is our goal and, admittedly, getting there can be challenging. We are so very busy these days, multi-tasking and running about, that we don't seem to take the time to delve into what God truly means to us or how that Presence is designed to show up. We travel the world, we frequent the mall, we stuff our closets with new items, and we buy more objects to make our lives easier, more improved. We look for the Ah-ha moment in coffee shops, seminars, on cruise ships and in bars. Repeatedly we chant, pray, beseech yet find we are on a treadmill going nowhere.

Frustratingly, nothing happens in our daily life to change where we are headed, or ever will, until we make the pure and true connection with God. Goldsmith tells us, *"In the presence of Sprit which is released when you touch the center of your being... matter and mind both become servants and tools."*

We'd much rather bargain with God or plead with God than fully understand what God is and what God isn't. We need to stop and refocus our attention on the greater goal and conscious conviction of the Presence of God within. We must stop and use the tools we have been given.

Joel Goldsmith writes, *"Having the assurance of the Divine Presence within you, you need nothing and nobody in this world."*

Our first goal then, is to convince ourselves, and hold impenetrable within our consciousness, that God is All there is. God is the tsunami and God is the sunlight. God is the diamond and God is the carbon. God is also the power and the pressure than turns the carbon into a gem. Our task, if we are to have true conviction of the One and the Infinite, is to understand that God is as much the lost child on the milk carton as It is the Iron Chef on the Food Network.

Having an understanding of God and living with Conviction are two different things. There are no shortcuts to arriving at this place of inner knowing. None of us can buy this awareness; it is not tangible; we cannot grow it in a window box, we cannot borrow it, or bake it, but we can establish it and prove it. We must have the assurance and ultimately the Conviction, that God, being the Living Power in and through everything, lives inside of us.

When we are sitting alone, when we are mentally quiet, when we put all of our distractions aside and turn deeply within, there, we can experience our Oneness with God; it is solely up to us. This experience of God is not going to come while we are too busy to make time for Divine communion, or too occupied with the have to's in our agenda. It will occur when we make room for God to pay us a private visit. We cannot ever forget; God is always in us and working through us. There isn't a time when God is not within.

When we make the time to connect to that Presence, we actively invite and welcome It into our *conscious* awareness and that's what makes all the difference. Having God within is one Truth but allowing the *experience* of that Presence to flood our consciousness is quite another.

When conscious awareness happens, heaven and earth meet. The alchemy of this convergence alters our lives forever. From this point on we cannot do anything except operate as the Presence of God, because we have invited It in, experienced It at the innermost core of our being and our hearts have responded to the dynamic, all-encompassing Presence of the Invisible power. We have sanctioned It and allowed It to be personal. At the level of personalization, the Power is unleashed, and we have mastered step one of *Supreme Healing.*

We are now certain; we have achieved Conviction. The Power of God may be impersonal; but the Presence of God within us is extremely personal and private; in fact, it is quite sacred. This intimate awareness is our purest experience of Grace.

We can return to the practice of deep communion as often as we choose. The real beauty of this experience is that it only has to happen once for our awareness to shift; we begin to think and act on a new plane. And, once we have had that experience, like a tattoo, it lasts forever.

Knowing God may be easier than you think. We trip over the word "power" and we believe it to be something external to each of us. The silly little secret that has kept many of us unhappy is that power by its very nature is within, not outside ourselves. Consider electricity for a moment. Where does it reside? It's not in the switch, or the lamp, or the light bulb; it's the invisible current that travels along the wire *to* the switch, the lamp and the light bulb. The power of electricity remains invisible and yet it lights up the night.

The word *power* originates with the French word *poeir* and perhaps rooted earlier in the Latin word *potere* from which we also get *potent*. Both words mean *having the ability* or *being able*. In the strictest sense of the word power conveys the concept of potential, of energy waiting to be put into action and it implies *by us*.

The root of the word suggests that with power we have the aptitude to *do* something. We possess the invisible essence, i.e. the power, to make something happen. We use our power, not our force, to generate transformation; in this case, our healing.

We must not try to force God into action through our mental channels. It does not work if we try to make a deal with God. *"If you do this for me; I'll do this (thing I know I should have been doing all along...) in return."* It does not work if we try to bribe God, *"I'll give up X if you'll do Y"*. It does not work when we try to negotiate with God, *"I'll give this much if you'll give that to me."* It does not work if we taunt or petition God, *"Look how good I've been, surely I deserve this."* It does not work if we threaten God, *"I'll do something really bad if you don't come through for me."*

Repeatedly we make the mistake of thinking that God must *do* something for us. There is nothing whatsoever personal about the activity of God. Nothing. Do you think that God would do more for you than for me? There is no such quality of God that would reward one and punish another; nothing that would make anyone of us better, more affluent, healthier or wiser than the next person.

You cannot use God like a fix-it tool and then put It back in the closet for the next time you need a repair. God is not your convenience store for a midnight miracle when you need filling up. You cannot pray to God and have God show up on your doorstep to do your bidding. Nor can you pray to God to make something happen. God is much smarter than that.

You must convince yourself that God does not dole out justice, punishment or rewards. And God is not a handy man that will *fix* things in your life or the world. God is not your employee, your attendant, your best friend, your servant or your enemy. God is God.

You might be under the impression that God wins games for the Lakers or the Celtics. But God doesn't. Instead, God moves through, and with, each member of both teams as a co-creative force, and the manifestation of the awareness of that co-creation is what ends up on the scoreboard. Some years produce the human form of winning scores; other years have results that do not demonstrate the winning side of the game. But the co-creative action is still *in play* just the same, and all of the time. God does not now, and never has, chosen the winning side. God is fully present on both teams, in and as the winners and the losers. The winners just played harder and believed more in today's game than the other team. God is neutral.

Joel Goldsmith explains how God works this way: *"The activity of God is like light touching darkness. It does not do anything whatsoever to the darkness: it does not heal it, correct it, change it or remove it. It just reveals that there is none. That is what the activity of God is like. In healing it does not heal a disease: it just reveals that there is none."*

I think that athletes and celebrities who get up and thank God for their awards are ill informed. I live for the day I hear an Academy Award Winner say, *"I accept this award tonight of behalf of me and the God within. I recognize that I am a unique expression of God in the form of me. Tonight, I celebrate the manifestation of power and co-creation between me and Spirit. And I thank the One God that lives, breathes and votes in the form of you. Together, we are Creation and I am grateful for knowing that."* [20] Now *that's* conviction and the complete Truth.

Goldsmith gives us this thought, *"Healing depends completely on your ability to make yourself completely conscious that God is the only reality, the only Power and the only Law there is. If you believe that anything exists outside of the One Power, then you are affirming duality and living in the illusion created by our human minds. We change our entire world when we look out at it and realize that it is only an effect, therefore it holds no power."* [21] When you have this experience of God there are no words, no rules just an experience than can barely be described, if at all. One moment you may be just like every other mortal and the next; you are transformed.

That's the way healing happens. It comes as the result of a complete and total connection with the Infinite in a way that surpasses all others that precede it. All that has occurred is that Spirit has come into manifestation. The affluence of God has overcome the carnal and transformation is experienced.

---

[20] Author

[21] Joel Goldsmith, *Invisible Supply*

Conviction comes to us as a gift of Grace. It arrives without fanfare, silently, and as gentle as a fog creeping in over an amenable seashore. Conviction outflows from our direct experience of Grace. It emerges simultaneously when we take the time to set aside our human activities long enough to reach a state of communion with God. It is the process of bringing our minds to a place of stillness where thinking is transcended, and the soul is allowed to receive the experience of the Infinite effortlessly.

Once we have experienced this enlightenment, our healing play unfolds according to a new set of rules. We act from spiritual guidance and not the narcissism of our past. (Everybody has a touch of narcissism; it is the human way of the ego prior to experiencing unification with God; we *can* get over it.)

A 14th century English mystic wrote in *The Cloud of Unknowing* that we must have discernment, not knowledge. No one can ever reach God through knowledge. *"God can only be attained when the altitude of consciousness is reached where the mind is at rest and the soul can receive the things of God."* Conviction, then, is an altitude of consciousness, a place above the activity of earth, where we meet the Creator on the Creator's own turf; a place of serenity, where the mind is purposely numbed into stillness, the heart is flung open and the soul embraces the Living, Vital, Presence of God.

But what if we have trouble getting to the moment of Conviction, how do we open up and let the light in?

I use a variation on the theme of the familiar *"Ask, Seek, Knock"* quotation from the Bible. The King James Version reads: *"And I say unto you, ask, and it shall be given you; seek, and ye shall find; knock, and it shall be opened unto you."*[22] When you want healing but your throat is sore from asking; when you have sought the path and your personal GPS is exhausted, and when you have knocked your knuckles raw, I say unto you, *"Quit! This is not working."* If you are not convinced, and cannot yet acknowledge consciously and passionately, in every cell of your body, mind and heart that God is right where you are, then you need to get busy and start practicing. You might want to try my approach: it's the **ASK** shortcut.

ASK stands for *"Assume Spirit's Knowledge."* Consider two meanings of the same words: Assume that Spirit is Knowledgeable and knows all, including what's on your mind and in your heart; and *Assume* that God's knowledge is your knowledge, too. In other words, you accept that since Spirit knows, so do you. Then your only task is to let it come forth *through* you. The act of assumption is a positive mental action.

Your mind connects the dots between God and yourself and you become aware there is no division between, but a unity. If God is all there is, and God is all Knowledge, it follows that if God is in you all the time, then all of the Knowledge of God is there too. Reasonable? Logical? Yes, and above all, true.

---

[22] Matthew 7:7, *King James Version*

The times I'm buried in a myriad of problems and I mistakenly believe they are mine alone to solve, I remember to **ASK** and *Assume* **Spirit's** *Knowledge.* It all comes back to me in that moment and I am able to down-stress, remember who *I am,* and proceed with a combination of the experienced knowledge I have earned, plus the spiritual knowledge that is embedded by Spirit. Suddenly, nothing appears as a mountain any longer and the journey across the mole hill, that felt like a mountain, becomes much more pleasant. When I reconnect with the Presence and Knowledge of God within me, I know that there isn't anything we can't solve together.

One of the best ways you can make room for God and increase your Conviction is by surrounding yourself with everything positive. I mean every detail. Every piece of art in your home should speak to you of empowerment. If it has a dark past, or creates a negative feeling in you, sell it or give it away. If you have furniture from past relationships that drags you down emotionally; release it, too.

Take an inventory of your home, room by room, and your workplace, also. Keep *only* the items that support your self-esteem, that bring you joy, that empower you to be who you say you are. Get rid of everything else that is tainted with a negative thought, memory or feeling and you will see how rapidly your home becomes a sanctuary of spiritual support. Reduce unnecessary clutter so that the life of Spirit can fill your home.

Every item in your home reflects your consciousness. You can make sure it mirrors what you want your life to be. Design the set of your spiritual play to send out the precise messages you want to express about your inner life. Allow the outer trappings to be an expression of your inner, personal world.

As in the action of a play, when the central character has *"the"* moment of illumination, everything in the plot, from that point on, is altered; it affects the outcome of the story, the fate of the characters, the dynamics of the action and the world they live in. You can consciously create *"the"* moment in your life by clearing the pathways so there is no blockage to your fulltime connection with God.

Conviction is ultimately concerned with the establishment of our world of belief. It sets the scene for the rest of our healing. When we have conviction, everything changes: we speak differently, we think with a fresh mind set, we act according to a higher order, and we love from a purer connection.

Rather than trying to get God to do something for us, how much more productive for us, and spiritually fulfilling would it be, if we were completely convinced that God is not a person who must do something for us but rather that God is just all there is. God is the Creative Force and we must learn how to allow It in and to use it in our lives if we are to change anything. The heart and soul of a life fueled by conviction is the inner experience of God.

Our ultimate goal is to reach the center of our being, and to be convinced of its Presence. From this center point out we have everything we need to improve upon a human or a spiritual condition.

With this Conviction, no situation can be too difficult, no person can overcome us, and we have a light within that guides us through the darkest hours and out of the most frightening of places. First, we must believe, and then we can move into true healing.

"(An) idea will find objective form in the outer world of the one who holds to it with conviction. It must first become established in the conscious mind. It will then transmit itself into a subjective embodiment and when this happens success will become habitual."[23]

[23] Ernest Holmes, *The Science of Mind*

Chapter Five

_____

Connection: The Second Act in Healing

"When you can listen to yourself, you can heal yourself."   -
                            Ceanne Derohan

In the previous chapter we established Conviction as our opening act in the Three Act Play of healing. Conviction is our concrete belief in the mind set (subconscious, organized pattern of thought and belief) that God is the reality in which we live. We positioned it as the center of our world. We also established the idea that the plot action develops according to our Mind Set.

Joel Goldsmith reminds us, _"If you hold in your consciousness that God is the only Source of your supply, you will always have your supply made evident to you even before you need it."_[24] Before you even think about it, God is there, poised and ready for action in your life.

Act One defines our world, the condition of it, establishes our mind set, the characters involved and the direction in which we are headed. Act Two develops the action, divulges more of the characters' traits and, through the mechanism of the plot line, reveals the challenges they face. Choices are presented; the decisions the characters make, scene by scene, will determine the final outcome.

_____

[24] David Hawkins, _The Eye of the I_

In Act Two of our healing adventure, we face our moment of Truth. As we set aside the cloak of the seeker, we open ourselves fully to the realization that God exists within us, as us; powerfully and potent. God is closer than our breath. God is deeply rooted within us that God reveals the Truth of who we really are, if we listen and pay attention. In this step we summon the humility for inner revelation and allow it to bring forth the wisdom that emanates from the Presence within. We *connect* to it.

Thinking about God, speaking about God or chanting mantras about God cannot bring us closer to healing any more than thinking about a symphony makes us a classical composer. We will remain frozen within the constraints of the human mind until we are able to make contact with the Spirit within to the point of actual realization. When it comes to healing we are the drum and not the drummer because we hold the totality of the music within.

To graphically explain how and where Connection occurs, we use the symbol of *Supreme Healing*:

Supreme Healing

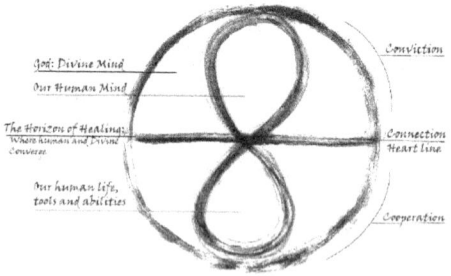

In this symbol the entire circle represents God as All There Is. The infinity sign within the circle symbolizes there is no time or place where that Power and Presence is not. The upper part of the circle is accepted and individualized by our Conviction of that belief. The top loop of the infinity sign represents our human mind within the Mind of God. The bottom loop represents our human experience within the Life of God.

The line in the middle represents the point where mind converges with the body. We call this the Horizon of Healing, it is our heart line and it is the very place where heaven and earth, the Divine and the finite meet. It is the horizon where simultaneously we connect, converge and heal. The bottom half of the circle represents our human experience and the reality we create by using the combined power of our mind and the Mind of God.

The goal of *Supreme Healing* is to consciously arrive at the realization and unification of all of these elements. We want the Power of the Divine Mind within us to support what our conscious human mind declares, and we want to utilize all of the tools from the steps we have learned to assist us in reaching our goals. Since our goal is healing, we work towards that goal where mind, body and heart converge; at the point we have already established, where the human connects with the Divine.

Let's return to our play analogy. Once the writer has established the world of the play, the players begin to speak and function in their roles according to the plot.

The actions and blocking are the same from performance to performance because the author has pre-determined what the outcome is; she has chosen the words and actions that most illustrate her point. The onstage dialog and action merely furthers the intention of the playwright. The author writes with a specific goal in mind, a lesson, a moral, or a truth as she constructs the ebb and flow of her intellectual design.

The entire play revolves around the author's message and all actions and dialogue are created to support this. The place of connection in a play is the moment when the audience gets the point. When the mind of the author, using the actors as vessels of communication, conveys a universal truth and the audience resonates with it, that's the moment of Connection. Every effective play ever written has such an *Ah ha* moment.

Our play analogy mirrors our Connection to the Mind of God. The convergence of the two seemingly separate entities, the visible and the invisible, lift their veils and in an instant they are experienced as One. That is the message of our spiritual healing play. We become enlightened at the heart line where the merger occurs.

It is the moment of spiritual jaw-dropping when we feel the Presence in our every cell. Electricity sparks and, striving for healing, we embark on this journey to acquire the moment of enlightenment, the *Ah ha!*, and fulfillment.

The quest ceases when we reach illumination and a deeper expression of life begins. For some the journey can last a lifetime; for others it can happen in an instant. The choice is ours. Our participation requires only the willingness of an open mind and heart.

One of the means by which we are able to reach inner knowing is by seeking to cultivate a climate of living in Grace. Joel Goldsmith tells us, "*The moment we turn from the human to the spiritual, it is inevitable that the Spirit will take over.*" Healing never begins at the human level of the problem or the condition; it originates at the Divine level of Power and Supply. Our job, if we want to heal, is to create the territory for the connection; the merging of our human awareness and the Divine Power within.

How and when we reach that point of Connection varies with each individual. There are many ways to attain inner knowing.

We have many tools that we can use to establish the atmosphere and the setting for the mystical convergence. Some of us have already had the experience of Connection and may simply need to recall it or recreate it. Others, who want to establish a direct method to connect the Divine and the human, can choose from a variety of methods. Some may choose meditation, which certainly works to clear away the debris of human thought and lay the field open for a comingling of Divine Mind and human matter.

Hypnotherapy is also an avenue that can be used to reach the inner stillness required to meet the inner healer. There is also a third way to reach awareness of the other side of healing which we will discuss later in the chapter.

Meditation Techniques

Let's consider the tool of meditation first. If you are already skilled at meditation then you may not feel the need to read this next part, but if you want to develop or enhance your meditations, or your ability to meditate, please read on.

Although many variations are available, there are basically just two types of meditation: Linda Chrisman writes, "*Concentration meditation practices involve focusing attention on a single object. Objects of meditation can include the breath, an inner or external image, a movement pattern (as in tai chi or yoga), or a sound, word, or phrase that is repeated silently (mantra). The purpose of concentrative practices is to learn to focus one's attention or develop concentration.*"[25]

The word meditation comes from the Latin word *meditari* which means *to concentrate*. When you engage in Concentration Meditation you begin by focusing your concentration on your breath or watching a flame, staring at an object, or using a mantra for the specific purpose of stilling your mind from the activities around you and allowing it to place all of its attention on a single thing.

At first you may experience a wandering mind and feel like you are pulling an overly active child back into line every other moment. If you do, it's okay. This practice requires focus, discipline and becoming familiar with the technique. No one ever drives a stick shift smoothly the first time.

---

[25] Linda Chrisman, *Meditation* http://www.answers.com/topic/meditation

In a short amount of time your techniques will grow stronger. As you work your concentration muscles more the process becomes easier, you relax more quickly, your level of consciousness deepens more rapidly, and you slip into a state of peace more easily.

In this type of meditation, you allow the object of focus to harness your conscious mind and you use it as the probe to bore through the incessant chattering of the mind to reach the desired state of relaxation and stillness. You want to achieve a state of mental neutrality, where nothing dominates, nothing intrudes and everything in your body, mind and heart is focused as one.

The goal of meditation is to become still as that moment in the winter forest when the last snowflake has fallen and there isn't a footprint in sight. You picture the moon as it softly rises over the horizon and darkness spreads its cloak against the sky; there is nothing present but God. In your inner garden, not even the planted seed makes a noise.

Chrisman continues her description of the second meditation technique,

"Mindfulness Meditation practices involve becoming aware of the entire field of attention. The meditator is instructed to be aware of all thoughts, feelings, perceptions or sensations as they arise in each moment. Mindfulness meditation practices are enhanced by the meditator's ability to focus and quiet the mind."[26]

---

[26] Ibid

Unlike Concentration Meditation, Mindfulness Meditation is initiated by *increasing* your awareness of what you are thinking, feeling, sensing, and seeing.

Your mind pans the room like a camera becoming aware of all that is outside of you and then, one by one, skillfully, you bring those impressions inside. You are the *stage manager* of your meditation. You quiet the house before the performance. One at a time, you begin to dim the lights of your mental activity. As you quiet the mind and still the soul, you fall deeper and deeper under the spell of the inner playwright. One by one, outer distractions release you from their grasp and melt away from your awareness, until the only thing that is left is a feeling of expectancy.

It is the moment in the theater when the lights have dimmed, you cannot hear a whisper in the house, and there is intense anticipation for the rise of the curtain. Here, in the theater of your soul, enlightenment awaits. When the curtain rises, action is commenced, and convergence begins.

You may be familiar with different styles of meditations. There are many: one site claims 108 different modes of meditation.[27] There are fifty types of meditation in the Buddhist practice, and over one thousand in Tibetan meditation.

There are more active forms of meditation, as well. The Sufis whirl and dance to reach a state of ecstasy; their physical abandon catapults them into a state of trance where they experience the blending of the two worlds.

---

[27] http://www.meditationsociety.com/108meds.html

Shamans often chant and dance in their meditations. There are an infinite variety of methods. Once you have determined what works best for you, use that.
In addition to Concentration Meditation and Mindfulness Meditation, I would like to mention one other form of meditation: Unintentional Meditation.

Have you had the experience of being in the shower and having creative ideas flood your mind? Or have you been in the midst of a project like mopping the floor or hoeing the garden and suddenly received an inspiration? What you've experienced is the result of an *unintentional* type of meditation. The mind has been focused on the actions of the body and engaged at only a shallow level of concentration and because of this the mind is in a receptive state, a state where ideas and inspiration propagate. When you are in one of these states the mind is at ease; it is not being taxed with math problems or defensive driving or putting together complex ideas.

Your mind is simply functioning at the lower level of awareness that is required to support the rote activities of the body and not much more. Think of it as mental concentration being loose and carefree.
These are the ripe moments when the invisible world can easily present itself. The mind is not bouncing around, chattering to itself, measuring, counting, justifying or solving anything in particular, it's just going along *dum de dum* and humming a familiar tune.

Divine Mind seems to love it when the human mind is dialed down a notch or two, as in *otherwise engaged*. Spirit can slip right on in and supply the answers, pop in a few new ideas, and stir the creative soup. The next time you are sweeping the patio, mopping the floor, digging a hole, or scrubbing the tile in the bathroom, think of it as an opportunity to receive insights from the invisible world.

Whichever form of meditation you choose, your ultimate goal is to reach a place where your conscious mind is distracted. The gear you want your mind to be in is neutral. The goal is to have no conscious thought dominating your mind, only a tranquil, open field primed for the arrival of something beyond the norm. In this state of silent expectancy your pulse rate slows, your mind is eased, and your heart is impartial.

Meditation in its variety of forms can result in that state easily and effortlessly if you just let it. How you choose to reach this state is up to you.

Hypnosis

Hypnosis is yet another method wherein you take yourself, or allow another person to lead you, into a trance state. Dr. Linda Joy Rose, a leader in the field of hypnosis, says: *"All hypnosis is self-hypnosis. You go into a trance many times a day whether you believe in hypnosis or not. The goal here is to use these natural states intentionally rather than be used by them."*[28] Dr. Rose believes that there are collective qualities to intentional hypnosis and the more frequently you induce the state, the deeper you will go each time.

---

[28] Linda Joy Rose, *Your Mind: The Owner's Manual*

If you want to engage in intentional self-hypnosis you may want to make a tape or a CD with your own voice that you can listen to and follow.[29] That MP3 or CD would contain four levels:

> 1) Centering and deep breathing through a progressive relaxation.
> 2) Deepening of the trance through guided imagery.
> 3) Connecting with Spirit - installing a switch.
> 4) Returning to full consciousness.

Preparing an MP3 or a CD helps you remain focused for the length of your altered state. You may want to write and design your own personal script and record it yourself. Here are some guidelines and a few sample scripts to follow.

Centering:

The purpose is to guide yourself into relaxation. Speak much more slowly than you normally would and pause frequently. You want to create an atmosphere of relaxation for yourself, not a pep rally. My suggestion is to rehearse a few sentences, record them and play them back. Your own sense of rhythm will tell you how slow or fast you need to read. At first you may be surprised that you *feel* you're speaking slowly, when in reality, you are reading quite fast. Try a test run and judge for yourself.

---

[29] My Prerecorded CD is available for you at www.spiritualgenius.com

Following is a sample script for you: (Words in parentheses are instructions to the reader for recording. (Pause) indicates that the reader should wait before going on to the next thought. If you have someone else read the script, it should be read in the second person:

"Begin to feel all of the tension melt away and leave your body. "Begin by taking three long, deep breaths. Inhale through the nose and out the mouth. Breathe in (pause 3 seconds) and.... breathe out (pause 3 seconds). Again, inhale (pause 3 seconds) and ...exhale (pause 3 seconds). Once again, big deep breath, in (pause 3 seconds) and.... let it go (pause 3 seconds). (Speak slowly) I begin to feel all of the tension melt away and leave my body. I allow each breath to take me into relaxation. Each breath relaxes my body and each breath takes me deeper and deeper into relaxation. I feel the muscles in my head and neck relax. I feel the tops of my shoulders relax. All of the tension simply melts away. (Pause) As I breathe, I relax even more and more deeply focusing on each relaxing breath I take.

(Continue speaking slowly) My arms begin to relax and release any tension, any resistance. (Pause) My hands and fingers completely and totally relax. (Pause) My chest relaxes more and more with each breath. (Pause) My abdomen relaxes. (Pause) My hips and buttocks relax. (Pause) Breathing now even more deeply as the relaxation continues down my legs. (Pause) The tops of my thighs relax. (Pause) The backs of my legs relax. (Pause) My knees relax. (Pause) My shins relax. (Pause) My calves relax. (Pause) My ankles relax. (Pause) The tops of my feet relax. (Pause) My soles relax. (Pause) And my toes completely and totally relax. (Pause 5 seconds.)

Take another deep, deep breath and slowly, release it. (Pause) Feeling now completely relaxed and totally at ease I release any last little bit of stress or tension that may be holding on. I breathe in ....and I breathe out.... letting go of anything that is not perfect, complete and total relaxation.

2) **Deepening:**

You will want to continue with your recording using a script similar to the one below: Remember to speak slowly and pause often, allowing time for the mental reply.

I imagine now my perfect, ideal setting. The place on earth, or in the universe, that makes me feel the most secure, the most beautiful, the most relaxed and happy. (Continue slowly) I Picture it in my mind and allow the scene to reveal itself around me (Pause) When I have that mental picture in my mind I allow myself to notice the temperature. Am I feeling warm? Is it cool? Is a breeze blowing? Is there a mist? Is it clear? What is the temperature? (Pause) Is it sunny? Cloudy? Overcast? Raining? (Pause) What time of day is it? (Pause) I take a moment to smell the air. The aromas I detect are.... (Pause) What season is this? (Pause) What colors are around me? (Pause) What is underfoot? Am I on a path? Grass? Bricks? Pebbles? Stones? Roadway? (Pause) Moving forward I can see in the distance a clearing. (Pause) I walk along the pathway to the clearing. (Pause) I see a body of water off to my left. (Pause) I follow the path to the water's edge. (Pause) I notice a bench by the water. I sit on the bench and just take in the view of the water. (Pause) I look all around me and I see the beauty of this spot. (Pause) I am completely comfortable, relaxed and feeling very happy. (Pause)

Off to the right side is a boat, moored at the edge. I notice the colors of the boat. (Pause) I walk towards the boat and I climb in. I am safe and I release the boat to move out into the center of the water. (Pause) I relax even more and lie down in the boat, supported by the soft pads in the boat, and, comfortable in my body, I completely relax and feel safe. (Pause) The boat rocks gently back and forth...to and fro.... gently moving side to side with the easy movement of the water. (Pause) Gently rocking now, side to side, tenderly moving, easy and slow. I feel myself relax even deeper and deeper as the gentle swaying of the boat continues. In this place and in this moment I feel as safe as I have ever felt.... as relaxed and happy as ever before..... And completely relaxed.

The boat and the water support my body and I fall even deeper into a state of relaxation. (Pause 10 seconds)

Now that I am completely and totally relaxed, I feel at peace. I am in complete harmony with all my parts and I allow myself to receive. I open my mind and my heart to welcome in the Presence of God, and I listen. (Pause 40-50 seconds)

Continuing in a state of complete relaxation and trust, I listen even more deeply to what is being said. (Pause 40-50 seconds or longer if you wish)

Information is being conveyed to me in thought, words and pictures. I continue to receive. (Pause 30-40 seconds or longer if you wish)

3) **Installing a switch**:

In this step you will confirm your connection and affirm your truth. You will place in your subconscious the statement and the realization of the perfection that you are; the ever-unfolding mirror of God that you always have been. By flipping an invisible *switch* in your mind, you will be able to return to this state of Grace and Connection at will. The following script shows you how to do that.

Anytime I wish to return to this state, anytime I wish total relaxation and total communion in this state of Grace, I can simply say the words:_____
(Fill in your own Connection phrase. It can be a name, a color, a mantra, a favorite saying, a blessing, any short combination of words that you will remember easily and often.) Simply by using my Connection phrase: (repeat the phrase) I am able to return to this state anytime I please.

Taking another moment now,
I affirm:_____ __
(Create a short statement that is positive and reflects your deepest desires.)

Suggestions: I affirm that I am completely healed, perfect in mind body and heart. I am love, I am Spirit-filled, and I acknowledge that the Power of God works through me, as me and in me all of the time. (Pause)

4.) **Returning to full consciousness**. As wonderful as this state of relaxation is, you will need to come back into the real world at some point. The suggested script follows, or you can invent your own.

As I allow the Presence of Spirit to fill me, I know I can return to this place and time of connection any time I wish to. It is here for me, (Pause) waiting for me, all the time (Pause) I have only to say my Connection phrase _____(insert your phase) and I will be transported back into this state of relaxation anytime I desire.

I feel the boat rocking gently beneath me. (Pause) I smell the air. (Pause) I become more and more aware of my body as the boat drifts back toward the shore. (Pause) I feel the boat lightly settle and land on the shore. (Pause) I raise myself up and I alight from the boat. (Pause) I am standing beside the shore now and I notice the temperature and the light around me. I walk back to the bench and turn to have one last look at the water and the boat that took me on my inner journey. (Pause) My heart is filled with gratitude and I bless the water, I bless the boat and I fill up, overflowing with gratitude for this extraordinary Connection. (Pause) I am centered. (Pause)

I turn now and head back on my path, feeling completely refreshed, totally inspired and happy. I walk slowly and confidently as I head back into my life renewed in God's Love and Light.

As I count back from ten, I will be fully and completely restored to my conscious self. (Pause) (Slowly count back)
 Ten (Pause)
 Nine (Pause)
 Eight (Pause)
 Seven (Pause)
 Six (Pause)
 Five (Pause)
 Four (Pause)

Three (Pause)
Two (Pause) Feeling more refreshed now than I
ever have been, coming back into my body fully
and...
One. I open my eyes and I am completely and
totally awake.

Congratulations! You have completed your own journey into the state of Connection, the second step in *Supreme Healing* . Play the tape or CD as often as you like, connect as frequently as you want and make a new tape or CD if this one becomes *old* to you.

The Pendulum

In addition to meditation and hypnosis, you may want to try another way to achieve the state of Connection. Using this method, you remain fully conscious, but step slightly aside into an altered state of awareness as you use the pendulum as a tool to dig deeper into your subconscious, reveal the healing wisdom within you and listen to what is being spoken from the junction point at the heart line.

The pendulum is not used as a tool for invoking *outside* forces, but rather as an instrument through which your consciousness may express, much like a pen is the tool through which a writer reveals inspired thought, or the paintbrush the artist uses to express her inspiration. All that is required is a pendulum and the charts below. The requirements are simple and surprisingly easy, yet the connection is powerful.

For some the use of the pendulum may come quite naturally; for others there may be a need to set aside preconceived notions about its use. I suggest that you allow yourself the experience of this extraordinary connection with your own inner wisdom. The scientific laboratory work of David Hawkins PhD from 1978-1998 provided, "*Kinesiology for the first time exposed the intimate connection between mind and body, revealing that the mind 'thinks' with the body itself.*"[30]

In his experiments Hawkins discovered that the body can discern to the finest degree the difference between that which is supportive of life and that which is not. Use the pendulum to tap into your inner resource of wisdom. The body responds in pure Truth to the questions asked. You will discover the answers you seek using this process.

In the 1960's, American dowser, Verne Cameron, demonstrated his special dowsing talent to the U.S. Navy by successfully locating, on a map, every submarine in the Navy's fleet. He also located every Russian submarine in the world. Based on the demonstration, the CIA determined that Cameron was a risk to national security, and he was forbidden to leave the United States. If discoveries by a pendulum work for the Navy, imagine what it can do for you.

Directions

1) Find a quiet space where you can be alone for a period of time; thirty minutes to an hour is recommended.

---

[30] Ibid

2) You will need a chair and a flat surface like a desk or a table in front of you.

3) You will need a pendulum and the charts that follow in this chapter.

4) Sit up straight, place your elbow on the flat surface and hold the pendulum chain between your thumb and your middle finger, with the excess chain held up by your forefinger. If you are right-handed, place the pendulum in your right hand; if you are left-handed, place it in your left.

5) Hold the pendulum above the middle point of each chart, allowing the tip of the   pendulum to hang 1/4 to 1/2" above the chart.

6) Set your intention that the pendulum will indicate the Truth.

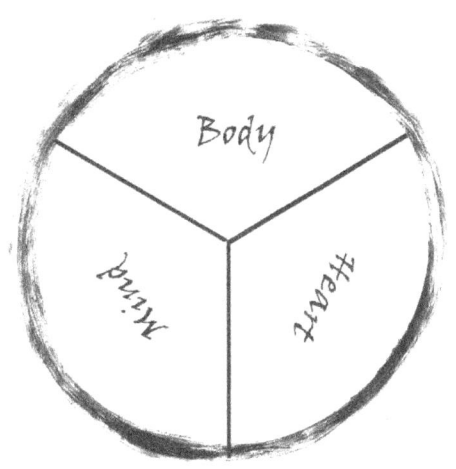

The purpose of this chart is to determine the location of the healing desired. Where is your healing needed most? If you are not sure *what* you need to heal in yourself, then mentally (consciously) step aside and allow your inner wisdom to tell you. Take a moment to release any tension you may feel from the day, relax your body and open your mind. Breathe deeply until your mind becomes a blank slate. When you are ready, follow the directions for this chart. Even if you think you know the answer, try it anyway.

Directions:

Hold your pendulum over the center of the preceding chart. Allow it to come to a resting position. Concentrate deeply on the following phrase and then speak the words aloud.

I am open to receive. Show me the area that needs healing. Show me the area now.

This process may take a moment. Until you become used to your pendulum and its physical activity, simply be patient and observe its action. In the beginning, the action of your pendulum may be wildly kinetic, or it may be shyly hesitant. Be patient. Stay with it. It will acclimate to your energy. Give it time to merge with you. Trust that your inner healer will communicate with you through this pendulum. Find the joy and the delight in this process; it takes time to get used to a new dance partner. Allow your rhythm to meld with the energy expressed by the pendulum. If you need to give it a start, do that. It's like priming the pump so the water can flow. It will reach its path of communication. And then, watch as it reveals your Truth.

The pendulum will ultimately swing to one of the sections of the chart: Heart, Mind or Body. Take note of which section it has chosen. When you know the region in need of attention for healing, move on to the chart that is specifically named for that area. If your pendulum reveals that healing is needed in your heart; then move onto the heart chart. If it indicates that healing is needed in your mind, move onto the mind chart. There are three charts for the next section; each chart corresponds to one of the areas in the first chart: Mind, Body and Heart. Before moving on to the second chart, remain in your meditative, still and silent mode, open and receptive and say:

I am open to you Spirit and ask you to lead me in the direction of my healing. Show me clearly which direction to follow.

Mind

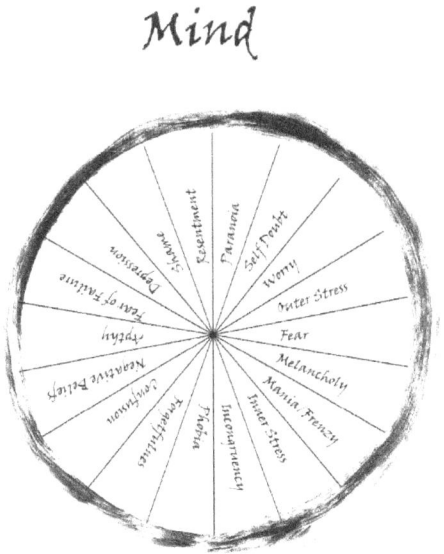

Body

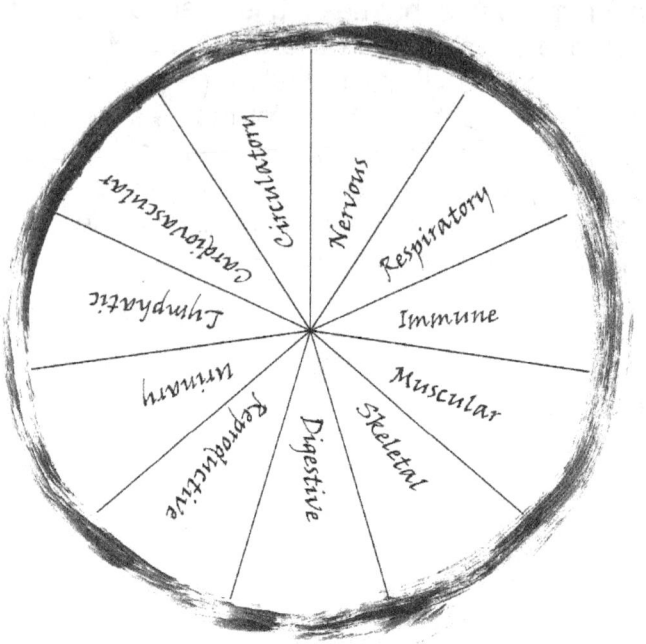

Heart

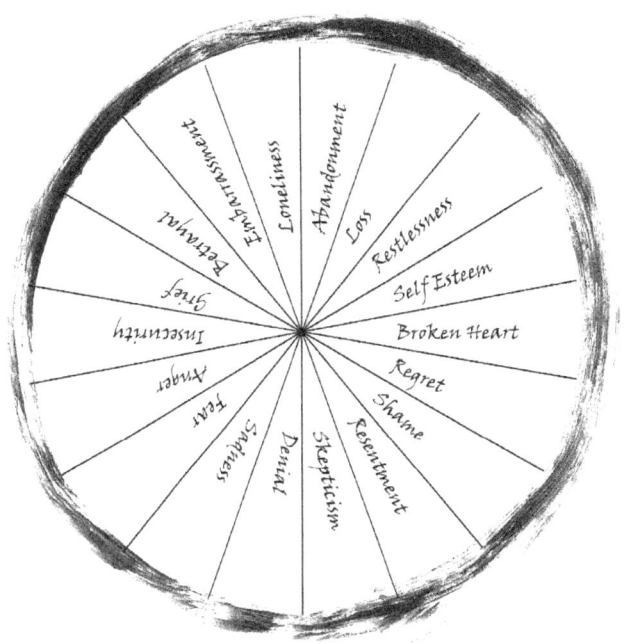

Turn to the appropriate chart, and when you are ready, repeat the process with the pendulum as you did with the first chart. Continue to sit very still, connecting deeply to your inner wisdom and allow the pendulum to lead you into the answer. The pendulum will guide you towards the specifics you need to know as you proceed along the process of *Supreme Healing*.

Your pendulum may swing back and forth equally in two directions and you may be confused as to which section it is indicating. Know that the direction of movement with the strongest and the most definite path is your answer. The pendulum naturally swings in both directions as it gains momentum, but it will ultimately give you a stronger line in one direction. Give it time; wait and watch for it.

The final step in the Connection stage is to ask your inner wisdom for the specific healing channels you will need to take. Use the final chart to lead you to the most appropriate channel to follow for your healing. You will simply ask:

Show me the channel I need to explore in order to bring this healing into my reality.

Allow the pendulum to guide you to the area where your answer lies.

Healing Channels

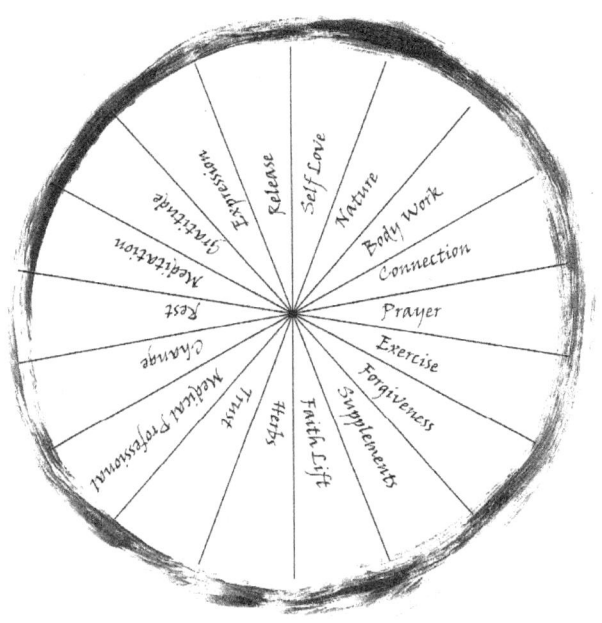

When you have completed your work and arrived at the answer in the final chart, *Healing Channels*, you have completed the second step, Connection, in *Supreme Healing*. You connected to your inner sage and you received answers. How does that feel to you? Are you more confident in your healing process? Be sure to live with the information for at least 24 hours. Consider what it means and what it requires of you. If you still have questions after 24 hours, repeat the process.

Often when something is new to us, we simply need to allow enough time to adapt. Think of it as an altitude adjustment. When you go 5,000 feet above sea level, your body takes a while to adjust; even bread flour rises differently. Grant yourself the time to acclimate to the process as well as the information. I suggest a nice long bubble bath, a steam or a Jacuzzi. Try the process again when you're fresh and clear. Connection is an important step and it may not be easy initially. You will get the hang of it if you stay with the process. Be gentle with yourself. If you need more time, take it. There is no rush in enlightenment.

With such a beautiful new tool at your disposal you have embarked upon sacred work. Cherish the process and use it with love and respect. It will provide you with the knowledge you need to improve and heal for the rest of your life.

In the world of the theater Act Two leaves us an unresolved set of circumstances and takes us to intermission. At this point, we have seen the characters encounter one situation after another and we leave them at the end of Act Two with a lot of information but an uncertain future. Which way will they turn? What will become of them?

How will they handle the next encounter? Will there be an opportunity for success or a setback? Will they fall in love? As with the play, the second Act of our healing journey, through Connection and exploration, leaves us with plenty of information. *Supreme Healing* occurs at the level where conviction meets connection. Cooperation is how we connect the two. How we deal with that information, and where we take it are the substance of Act Three: Cooperation.

Remember the clear light, the pure clear white light
from which everything in the universe comes,
to which everything in the universe returns;
the original nature of your own mind.
The natural state of the universe unmanifest.
Let go into the clear light, trust it, merge with it.
It is your own true nature, it is home.
         - Tibetan Book of the Dead

In closing this chapter, the words of Joel Goldsmith inspire us, *"You are not the actor; you are not the healer; the concern is not yours. You are relaxing yourself into Grace and Grace is going to do the work: you are merely going to be the instrument of Grace."*[31]

---

[31] Joel Goldsmith, *Invisible Supply*

Chapter Six

Cooperation: The Third Act in Healing

"I learned that healing and cure are active processes in which I myself needed to participate." Rollo May

We have gathered our information and received feedback from our inner healer in the Second Act of *Supreme Healing*, Connection. Using our playwriting analogy, Act Three of our healing play gathers all of the pieces together to reach the dramatic summation. It is time for the resolution and the climax. Everything up until now, every word, every character, every action of the plot in previous acts has built towards this ordained solution, conclusion and purpose. As in the theatre; so it is with our healing quest. All truth is revealed and brought into focus in the Third Act.

In *Supreme Healing* the Third Act is called Cooperation. Cooperation is defined as *all elements working together for a common purpose.* [32] In Act Three all that we have previously learned, studied, and all that has been revealed to us is gathered for practical use and application. When we fully cooperate with our body, mind and heart in the healing process, the synergistic trilogy of body, mind and heart comingle to manifest our desired results.

Exploring the concept of Cooperation, we begin with the mind in our healing trilogy.

Healing the Mind

---

[32] Webster's Dictionary

To attract our collective attention, advertisers and marketers use dramatic media campaigns to create national health scares. With few exceptions, diseases are labeled as *enemies* and, as a result we have created, the *War on Cancer*, the *Fight Against Diabetes*; simultaneously we *Combat Germs*, *Battle Breast Cancer*, and *Conquer Heart Disease*. The consciousness both individual and collective, that we create by going to war with physical conditions may be harming us more than the condition itself. When we are continually *bombarded* by terms that describe an opposition mentality, War, Combat, Fight, Disarm, Seize, Battle, those terms create opposing camps and adversarial relationships. Why would we do that?

Supreme Healing calls for cooperation with your condition no matter what it is. Unlike those who might tell you to ignore the fact of a disease, or to fight it, *Supreme Healing* requires that you embrace it first before you change it. Any disease is a perfect, whole and complete condition of something. It is merely doing its job and performing its function *as* the condition. It's working hard to be the best disease, germ, virus it can be. Give it credit for doing it well.

Initially it might seem strange or uncomfortable to honor a disease for its accomplishments; but there is a purpose behind the unfamiliar approach.

In the case of a disease or the condition we'd prefer not to have, we first appreciate it for simply being what it is: it has functioned as a whole, perfect and complete illness and we need to acknowledge it for having accomplished that much, very well.

The principle behind this appreciation for the *enemy* can be found in martial arts. In Aikido one is trained not to attack his opponent, but rather to come up alongside him and engage via strength, position and balance to overtake him. A joining of forces, called *"blend and enter"* occurs and the strongest *energy*, not the largest fist, dominates the situation. This is a mental as well as a spiritual practice where one *defends* by placing the opponent off balance.

If we *go to war* and *attack* our condition it will fight back harder. As in Aikido, *Supreme Healing* aligns with the condition, at the level of Cooperation, training it away from a negative path through the use of strength of persuasion, and not by engaging in an onslaught of warfare.

Consider the dynamic another way: if a guy in a bar throws a punch chances are strong that someone will return that punch with equal or greater force, in other words, fight back.

The same is true of disease. If you throw a punch in direct combat, the disease/condition will punch back even harder, as though it was fighting for its life, which it actually is.

The more successful and longer lasting approach is to ease alongside the disease/condition, discover what it thrives on, what feeds it, what promotes its advancement, and then intentionally weaken it, and steer it away from its supportive resources. *Cutting it off at the pass*, or preventing its supply to live and thrive, is far more effective, spiritually, than all-out mind/body combat.

Suppressing a disease or a condition with strong medicines is the same as going to war with it. We need to get to the root of it in order to heal it, not mask it or camouflage it.

In previous chapters discussing the process of healing, we have said that it requires Conviction, Connection and Cooperation to achieve *Supreme Healing*. To attain these three states, four key factors are necessary: belief, thought, mental imagery, and emotion. Conviction holds belief and thought, Connection establishes mental imagery, and Cooperation embraces emotion.

First and foremost is the importance of belief. *"The fact is that belief is the master key to healing, that the physical mechanisms of cures of disease, whatever their nature, make connections to the immaterial realm of the mind."* [33]

What we believe affects the quality of our healing. But how do we really know what we believe or how to change those beliefs if we discover we aren't achieving the results we want by them? It all boils down to self-examination. If you want to heal, you must begin with introspection. We can only change a belief by looking at it from a different perspective, adjusting our mind set and then believing that new idea. The first step is discovering what you really believe. If you want to know more about what you believe, you must look at your life.

Answer the following questions honestly:

> What are your priorities?
> Where do you spend your time?

---

[33] Andrew Weil, *Spontaneous Healing*

What do you spend most time doing?
What would you do if you didn't have to work?
What would you do if you didn't have any ties?
What would your life be if you didn't have
_____?
Where does your imagination take you when
you have a quiet moment?
Who or what inspires you?
Who or what do you want to get even with?
Name one thing that would solve all your
problems.
Finish this sentence:
If only

_____

_____

What makes you happy?
If you had one wish what would it be?
If you had a week to live what would you do?
If your life was perfect it would look like

_____

Describe your happiest memory.

_____

_____

Complete these sentences:

Money is_____
Family is _____
Work is _____
Friends are _____
Rest is _____
Relief is_____
I have _____
I need _____
I want _____
I am _____

The five most important things in my life are:

1 _____
2 _____
3 _____
4 _____
5 _____

The next step in discovering what you believe is to take out your pendulum and use the *Yes* or *No* method to answer the questions that follow. Hold the pendulum in your dominant hand and place it over a piece of blank paper. Steady it, center it, and ask the pendulum, *"Tell me which direction is Yes".* Allow it to swing in one direction or another. If it circles or doesn't move, wait for it to answer. Have patience. Once you know the *yes* direction, steady it and ask it, *"Tell me which direction is No."* Wait for it to respond. You may get a circle as a response. Allow it to circle and keep asking for a *definite* direction for *yes* and *no.* (You want *up and down* or *side to side.*) Once you are in tune with each other, ask the following *yes or no* questions and wait for each response.

Do I believe.....

in limitations
in mind over matter
a co-creative power within
the inherent goodness in humankind
disease is a punishment
evil is everywhere
in scarcity
some people are special/blessed/chosen
change is hard

in fate
healing is natural
the mind is separate from the body
only doctors can cure disease
in miracles
in self-power

Make a list of your answers. Now, using your
pendulum again, hold it over the following chart and
observe which way it swings. Let it tell you what you
secretly believe about yourself deep down.

Core Beliefs

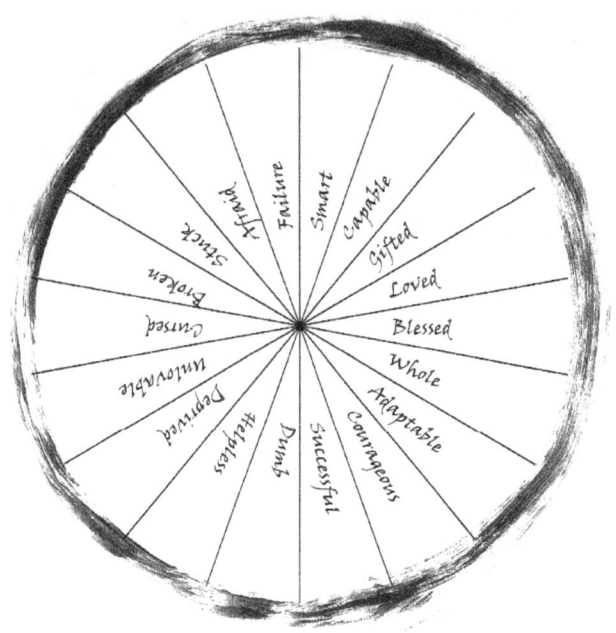

Follow up:

Were you surprised by any of your answers? Are there beliefs that you no longer want to have? Do you have a desire to change the beliefs that do not serve you? If so, there are Five Steps you can use to change any belief you want to. Use these steps often to create the new thoughts you want to have and hold in any area of your life.

First: Hold the belief you *don't want* in your mind.

Second: Change the belief to the belief you *do* want. Add color to your picture.

Third: Intensify that picture and make the colors more vivid.

Fourth: Bring that picture into your heart and fill it with love. Feel what it would be like to have, do or be what you are picturing. Make it personal.

Five: Let it go. Release the thought from your mind. Let it fly off into the ethers.

Firmly and absolutely, expect the change to occur.

When you have successfully inventoried your cache of beliefs, retained the ones you like, and replaced the ones you don't want with new ones that empower and increase you, it is time to move on to the next consideration.

Healing the Heart

"The belief that the spirit within us is capable of regenerating the physical body is based in truth. The Spirit can heal the body, the mind and matters of the heart."[34]

We count on our minds to research, determine, and act upon what is required in the realm of our physical healing, but the true key to complete healing rests in the heart. It is centered in forgiveness. Carolyn Myss says, *"In the end forgiveness is an act of release; surrendering the need for explanation."*[35]

[34] Carolyn Myss, *Defying Gravity*

[35] Ibid

How many times do we knock on the same door wanting an answer to *why* this happened or *why* it had to be me? *Surrendering the need for explanation* requires patience, perspective and humility. If we continue to hold on to the past by putting a leash around its neck, tugging on it and begging it to make sense, then we are lost. If we have a death grip on childhood pain, broken promises, personal betrayals, unresolved differences, deals gone sour then we have blocked our hearts against the flow of healing.

Forgiveness opens up our healing flow. It allows us to take on a characteristic of the Divine and exhibit compassion, first to ourselves and then to others. [36] *"Healing comes from gathering wisdom from past actions and letting go of the pain that the education cost you".*

The truth is that you don't have to go through years of therapy or endless hours of telling your story, you only have to decide to give up the need to know *why* and *how* something happened; accept that it did and get on with it. Release the need to ask *why me?* You could wait a lifetime for an answer.

I have a friend who lost her husband ten years ago. When she called me with the news she was very upset and sobbing. I had been the last person to leave a message for him on their answering machine, so I received one of the first calls about his death.

---

[36] Ibid

He had made a decision to end his life gracefully. He did not trust the illness that had invaded his body to allow him a departure with dignity. He believed, and surrendered to, the diagnosis that he was terminal and that he had a short time to live. As he did not wish to suffer painfully any longer, or put his wife through the agony, he took matters into his own hands and ended his life.

He prepared meticulously for his death so that no one close to him had the grim discovery of the final deed. He left loving reminders throughout the house of the happier days of his life and marriage. His was an elegant and graceful departure even if it was by his own hand and at his preferred timing and location.

After several days of intense grief, my friend was catapulted into planning his memorial. She never returned to her deep place of sorrow after her initial days of grief. Although they had been an extremely close couple, and she missed him desperately, she rapidly realized that she could not change the circumstances and bring him back. She chose, instead of being a victim of resentment or betrayal, to remember the love and to forgive him.

She never forgot him and all the joy they had together, but she released her attachment to the past and went on with her life. She was a great example to all of us. She never let the pain of her loss impede her progress and the path she was meant to follow. She forgave her husband and, in doing so, she also forgave herself, healed her wounds, and opened the door to the rest of her life.

Forgiveness is a key element of all healing, no matter how difficult it may seem or how intense the circumstances. Follow three steps to forgiving – you can make them as simple or as complex as you choose.

Step One:

Love and accept yourself exactly as you are in this moment. The past is over. Use the Three R's as your guide to self-acceptance: Repay, Repair, or Recant. Repay whatever you have borrowed or taken from someone else; Repair a relationship or a promise that you may have broken; Recant, or take back, anything hurtful you might have said or done directly or indirectly to someone.

Do what you need to do to stop feeling guilty about things that happened in the past. Once you have made the effort to amend, then accept what happened as having occurred because of the level of your experience and maturity at that time and move forward. If someone else continues to hold on to the past situation after you have made amends, simply allow them to do that; you can do no more. Once you repair, repay or recant, advance. Forgiveness can transform a misdeed into a gift. Accept what was, let it go, and begin to take a more active role in creating what will be.

Step Two:

Love and accept others. *"No kind word goes unnoticed. All is recorded in the field of consciousness."* [37]

---

[37] David Hawkins, *The Eye of the I*

Recall a time when someone gave you the benefit of the doubt or let you off the hook   for something. Do you remember how grateful you felt for that act of kindness? Perhaps it wasn't conscious kindness at all, but it was the result of the spiritual maturity of the other person who knew that people do the best they can, based on what they know, in any given situation. Understanding that although it may not have been what you would choose to do, or what you would want to happen, it was the best they could do in the moment. Kindness is a gift of the heart.

Kindness is a close cousin to forgiveness; forgiveness comes from a wise heart. Heart wisdom helps us to put into perspective the actions and intentions of someone else and give them the benefit of the doubt.

In one of her sermons on Mother's Day at SpiritWorks in Burbank, CA., Reverend Marlene Morris asked her congregation; *"What if the only gift you gave your mother today was to let her off the hook?"* You could hear the wheels tuning in the minds of the people listening. As popcorn explodes in a microwave, these thoughts were bursting like hot kernels in the minds of the congregants.

Among the popping thoughts were: *"Well I don't think I could go that far. After all, she…..." "Oh no, I couldn't do that."* And just as quickly as the frowns betrayed the resistant thoughts, there was a silent turnaround. Suddenly, and as quickly as the objections surfaced, new options opened up in the minds of the audience.

The thought kernels kept popping and protests magically turned into permission. New ideas emerged rapidly. Thoughts turned to, *"Why not?"* and *"That's a good idea."* And, *"I never thought of that."* or, *"Sure that could be a possibility,"* or *"It couldn't hurt to try."* The stagnant air suddenly blew fresh.

Reverend Marlene stood at her podium smiling and waiting while the machinations of thoughts went from negative to positive and the congregational minds transformed objections into acceptance. As soon as the audience caught on to what had just transpired, they broke into a soft and loving applause. They acknowledged her subtle "gotcha" and decided to play along.

What Reverend Marlene did that day was call them forth into a new paradigm and a new relationship with an old thought. This new perspective involved forgiveness and love. *"She did the best she knew how"* was the theme of the day, and in that hour many hearts were healed, and a multitude of tears shed. Most importantly the very question opened the channel for a new way of looking at the past so its gifts could be carried into the future and the scars left behind.

Those who had good feelings about their mothers were able to apply the same lesson to other situations and people. The example transcends time and personalities and translates to everyone and all circumstances.

Step Three:

"Spontaneous healing can be triggered by mental events and it can also be frustrated by habitual ways of thinking."[38]

Move your attention from the past to the present and into the future. Refuse to be held back by past thoughts, actions or conditions. Focus on tomorrow with all of the presence you have today. Become aware that you are a vehicle of consciousness and you are creating your future with every heartbeat. Let your heart select the musical score for your soul. Heart wisdom will guide you through the dark nights and into the light of a fresh beginning.

Get in touch with your heart wisdom by taking a moment in the midst of any challenging situation to give your heart a voice. If you want to shift the way you are thinking and feeling about something to access your heart wisdom, do the following:

1. Stop what you are doing: pull over if you are driving, turn off the computer, put down the phone, walk away from the confrontation, step aside, retreat.
2. Close your eyes and grab hold of what you are feeling.
3. Bring your heart up into to the situation and fill it with love.
4. Feel that feeling. Decide what your actions should be from this place, given what you really want.
5. Return to the situation and respond from your heart.

---

[38] Andrew Weil, Spontaneous Healing

This five-point system works every time. You will get the clarity you need, and you will act from the center of your heart when you take a moment to gain a new perspective. When you use the five steps, and you want the very best outcome, always follow your heart.

There is a classic story, well told by David MacArthur in *The Intelligent Heart*, of a Rabbi teaching love and appreciation to one member of his congregation. A man had become irritated with his wife's constant nagging and complaining, and he was thinking about getting a divorce. He went to see the Rabbi to seek advice. The Rabbi listened, noted the man's anger and, surprisingly, asked him if he didn't want to get a little revenge before divorcing her. The man, eager to get even with her for the years of misery he had suffered, asked the Rabbi how he might accomplish that.

The Rabbi told the man to pretend that he cared about his wife and to tell her that she was beautiful, thoughtful, and loving. The result, the Rabbi told him, was that when he divorced her in a few months she would feel the loss of such a great man; she'd realize that she could never get a man as wonderful as him, and she would feel deep remorse. The man was overjoyed at the idea of setting her up for such a fall. The Rabbi instructed him to tell his wife every morning that she was beautiful and to thank her profusely for everything she did, no matter how small. The fiendish plot appealed to the man greatly.

Sometime later the Rabbi ran into the man on the street and asked him if he enjoyed being single.
The man looked at the Rabbi with a good deal of surprise and said, *"What are you talking about, why would I want to divorce such a beautiful, thoughtful and wonderful woman?"*

He wasn't even aware of the change, the healing, that he had created by moving his thoughts out of the past and into a possible future; he just did what the wise Rabbi told him to do. In pretending to appreciate her, he eventually believed his own thoughts and moved up two letters of the alphabet from criticism to appreciation and changed both their lives.

Appreciation works both ways. It transforms the perspective of the appreciator and it alters the experience of the one being appreciated. The heart is capable of transforming any situation from one of agony into joy. It's a matter of perspective.

"What the people in the world actually want is the recognition of who they are on the highest level, to see that the same Self radiates forth within everyone, heals their feeling of separation, and brings about a feeling of peace."[39]

Healing the Body

"The body is not separate from the whole, but it is part and parcel of the universe and its survival is a function of the whole." David Hawkins

During a visit to the USA last fall, friends from New Zealand described how shocked they were to see the plethora of cold products advertised on our television stations. *"It's Cold and Flu Season"* the commercials announced as though it is a predestined epidemic that couldn't be avoided.

---

[39] David Hawkins, *The Eye of the I*

Advertisers of everything from cough syrup to cold medicine attempt to program our minds with the distinct fatalism that colds and the flu are unavoidable. Clearly, we better get to the store right away and buy their products to lessen the effects of the inevitable onslaught over which we appear to be powerless. In New Zealand there is no seasonal cold and flu television broadcast campaign, and interestingly, there aren't many cases of a cold or the flu.

When we give power to a thought, we give the thought permission to manifest as a condition in our lives. If advertisers announced, *"Welcome to the Season of Perfect Health"* might we not create health instead of colds? Goldsmith described it, *"The mesmerism of the world is such that succumbing to temptations becomes very easy. Each one of us may fall in a different way unless we consciously use every ounce of awareness we have to maintain and sustain our spiritual integrity."* [40] It takes work to stay conscious.

When Louis Pasteur said: *"The germ is nothing; the soil is everything,"*[41] he meant that the most important control we possess is over the soil. The soil we speak of here is the environment of our thoughts. In the form of thoughts, awareness, and material nourishment, we control what goes into to the mind and the body; hence we have dominion over what composes the loam of both.

---

[40] Joel Goldsmith, *Invisible Supply*

[41] *Deathbed admission of Louis Pasteur* to Antoine Bechamp/Claude Bernard

If you or someone else has put something in your soil that you do not wish to have there, you must remove it, change it or cleanse it. Just as the farmer tills his field and readies it for planting, you must prepare your mental, spiritual and physical soil for that which you *do* want growing in your life. Soil with plenty of nutrients, like a deep connection to Spirit, and healthy life-sustaining foods, create a climate of strength in the soil of the mind and body. Germs cannot thrive when they are overpowered by a healthy environment. Cooperation between the person and soil is the key to keeping out the unwanted invaders.

In the Hawaiian Shamanic tradition of cloud busting there is an exercise designed to keep the Shaman's mental and spiritual acuity sharp. The Shaman's focuses thought inside the cloud so as to become *one* with the cloud itself. Having made that connection, The Shaman *as* the cloud, *makes a decision* to break apart; the result is the cloud splitting off into two or more different directions.

Using this same technique on client's body, the Shaman goes *inside* the disease or condition, becomes unified with it at the mental level, and, as the disease, makes a decision to return to wholeness. The Shaman cooperates with the disease by joining with it and then overcomes it by changing its mind, altering its power base and dissolving it.

Cooperation with disease does not suggest weakness or giving in to it. Cooperation, in this case, is for the purpose of diagnosing, researching and then supporting the desired condition; while denying the undesired condition its resources. *"Only when your sickness becomes sick will your sickness disappear."*[42] Our goal is to identify and dis-empower the undesirable condition.

These are the directives for physical healing:

1) Diagnose the condition; gather input from many points of view and from different branches of healing.
2) Respond to your condition; do not react to it.
3) Your body is not a machine; it is a living, dynamic organism, with an ongoing, unlimited process of regeneration. respect that.
4) Treat your body like a saving account; store up resources.
5) Cooperate with your body and give it what it needs to serve your life's purpose.

1) *Diagnose the condition.*

Hippocrates gave us the basis for understanding the complex relationship between body and nature when he said, *Premium non nicer:* First do no harm. He also said: *Vis medicatrix naturae*: Honor the healing power of Nature. These statements are what the doctrine of Hippocratic medicine is based on.

---

[42] Lao Tzu, Tao Te Ching

Hippocrates believed that recognizing nature's inherent power to heal was the key to diagnosis. Defensive medicine must back everything up with lab experiments, but observational medicine uses intuition as strongly as it uses instruments. With careful observation, you can become your own physician. Diagnosis means *to discern: dia* refers to today and *gnosis* means knowledge. A diagnosis then, strictly speaking, is the discernment of today's knowledge. As with the seasons, that knowledge can change and vary with each rotation of the earth; with each new day.

Different disciplines use a variety of methods to reach the *diagnosis* of a condition. Western medicine relies on x-rays, blood work and MRI's; Eastern medicine is based on the flow of Ch'i (life force), temperatures, pulses, electromagnetic fields and the balance of yin/yan within the body.

Kahunas look to muscle tension and mental beliefs to determine the path to a cure or remedy of a physical condition. Vedic healers regard the importance of certain body types based on the preferences of the five senses and physical characteristics before settling on a cure. There are many different approaches and it is wise to research several options and professional opinions before choosing a route for healing.

During a recent visit to a homeopath, Dr. Gregory Manteuffel, accompanying a friend, I witnessed an observational intake. The physician asked many questions, "Tell me when your condition feels better, and describe the surroundings. Is it better or worse when you are in hot weather? Do you feel better in morning or at night; when you are hot or cold? Do you feel worse when it is raining, cloudy, or sunny? Do you prefer a salty or sweet taste? Do you prefer sour or spicy? Are you more tired in the morning or in the afternoon? Do you become forgetful when you are tired? Are you quicker to anger or quicker to forgive?"

The questions were not about the condition itself, but the *soil*, the environment, the physical and the emotional aspects surrounding the condition. Dr. Manteuffel told me, "I was exploring what were the characteristics of her vitality, or defense mechanisms - what stressed it, what characterized it, what brought about its downward spiral. These fingerprints lead me to my choice of what remedy would reverse this downward spiral and fortify the defense mechanisms by applying a medicinal force synergistic with the formidable power of her built-in self-healing vitality."

It was a fascinating experience because of the many levels and dimensions that were explored. The condition was not just assessed by blood tests, x-rays, cold facts and clinical summaries, Dr. Manteuffel was looking for context. He wanted to know how the condition reacted when exposed to different situations. As the situation changed, the condition might also shift and change. These were clues he used to determine a remedy that would act *with* the body to affect its own healing.

The questions made me think more deeply about the definition of *condition* than I ever had before. I began to see it in a context in which it interacted with many other facets of life. I began to see cause and effect interrelating on an even larger scale. I could see where an imbalance here or there might tip the scale and trigger a condition. As the comic Artie Johnson would say, "*Velly Intellesting.*"

Andrew Weil writes, "*Health for the Homeopath is a study of balance reflecting the divine harmony of nature: disease is a state of imbalance characterized by sets of symptoms peculiar to individual patients.*"[43] Health then is a state of perfect balance and the cooperation of bodily systems. The healthy body represents a state of balance between complementary and opposing forces of the universe.

Clearly, to demonstrate health, this balance must be restored.

You may select western medicine, eastern medicine or any variety of alternative and complimentary practices. The directive is to get more than one opinion. Each branch does not have all of the answers, so use them according to your own intuition. The more points of view you have, the more choices you will have to support your healing process. The ideal is a team composed of several disciplines that share information and work in a complimentary manner. If you don't have access to a center like that, create your own by gathering a variety of opinions.

2) *Respond to your condition; do not react to it.*

---

[43] Andrew Weil, Spontaneous Healing

Lao Tzu would tell us that a response is preferable to a reaction, as a response is in tune with the true way of life (Tao). He writes:

> "As the soft yield of water cleaves obstinate stone. So, to yield with life solves the insoluble."[44]

The master speaks to two issues: one of yielding and the other of following the natural path to healing. This is akin to the practice in Aikido of working with the energies that are present, and not against them.

Remember, there is nothing we have to defeat or conquer, just to persuade and redirect energy.

When we respond to the situation and do not react to it, we are in harmony with it and therefore in full Cooperation. By *responding* to a situation or a condition we take a larger view of it. We do not *react* in haste, on impulse, or out of the emotion of the moment. We consider the options, evaluate our position and then *respond* in accordance with our desired outcome. Response puts us in control of the effect.

The most effective healing emanates from working *with* the energies at hand; it is about restoring balance. When we respond, we reflect on the desired outcome.

---

[44] Lao Tzu, Tao Te Ching

We give ourselves time to assemble all of the pieces; consider a variety of options and move forward having made a decision based on the whole. Whole thinking is far more effective than grasping the first option based on scattered, unrelated, random thoughts. Don't settle for the first opinion; consider several, weigh all of the input and, from that assessment, formulate a multi-faceted plan for healing. Always take time to consider what is the most effective response to your findings and diagnosis (today's knowledge).

Often the healing process can require emotional as well as physical support. Whole thinking considers every layer of the human package. We have physical, spiritual, psychological and emotional considerations that come with our physical needs. Look to support all your facets during the process of returning to wholeness. The hidden source of the disharmony may surprise you.

3) Your body is not a machine; it is a living, dynamic organism, with an ongoing, unlimited process of regeneration.

Andrew Weil tells about interviewing a river specialist when he was in college. The specialist said, *"You can dump sludge into a river and up to a point the river can detoxify itself and remain in good health. But if you keep dumping sludge at some point you will exceed a critical level where natural purification mechanisms become overwhelmed and break down.*

Plants and beneficial microorganism die, and the river becomes sick. But the miraculous thing is that if you stop dumping sludge into the river, eventually the contaminates drop to a level where natural healing mechanisms revive, oxygenation increases, sunlight penetrates to deeper levels and the river cleans itself up."[45]

Not only is this the type of healing that happens in nature, it occurs in our human bodies as well. All of the vital circuitry and machinery is present. We just have to locate the switches which activate the healing process. How do we increase the helpful ingredients in our internal soil so that the body is able to resist the invaders? Consider these points:

The body wants to be healthy. Health is the natural condition of perfect balance that occurs when all the systems run smoothly, and energy circulates freely. When the body is out of balance it yearns to get the balance back. The body wants to be healthy because being healthy signifies the efficient and optimum operation of all systems.

The body always seeks to heal itself and, like nature, it has a built-in process. Sometimes we have to get out of the way and let it follow its own path to recovery. In some cases, patience may be the only medicine required.

---

[45] Andrew Weil, *Spontaneous Healing*

Healing is a natural power. Creation and recreation are part of the natural cycle of life and the essence of being alive. Healing is natural, but it requires energy to heal and that energy must be supplied so that the body can operate at optimum levels. We have the ability to supply the energy our body needs for premium efficiency.

The body is a whole and all of its parts are connected. The body is a unified functioning set of systems and each system complements and supports the next.

"Belief is carried through the nervous system to the site of the illness. The cardiovascular system plays a role in increasing blood flow or decreasing it. The immune system participates since it can produce specialized cells to attack and destroy foreign matter and remove diseased tissue and cells. The respiratory system is involved because it carries oxygen to the diseased part that brings it the molecules of life and strength to remove the unwanted matter.

The urinary system is involved because it carries dead matter out of the body; the circulatory system is involved because it distributes new cells to replace the dead or diseased ones and brings nutrients for its growth."[46]

All systems are interrelated and interdependent. If the ankle is crooked, it creates a knee problem which, in turn, creates a hip problem and so on. (see Appendix A for more information on systems.)

---

[46] Andrew Weil, *Spontaneous Healing*

There is no separation of mind and body. *"Belief is carried through the nervous system to the site of the illness."*[47] Every system is part of the whole. Beginning in the mind, belief affects every part of your body.

That's why is it crucial to understand what you believe and change the beliefs that do not support your health and wellbeing. Change your beliefs at the level of Spirit and you will change the substance and performance of your body.

There is no guilt in illness. Many books about healing place blame or want to deflect the cause for illness and disease to the emotional make-up or attitude of the ill person. I do not support any philosophy that makes a person wrong for having an illness.

It is the last thing anyone needs when they are in the midst of a health crisis or dealing with the dark elements of a painful condition.
When someone discovers something that is causing their system to be out of balance, what they need is compassion and support, not finger pointing and culpability.

In addition to our beliefs, our health is impacted by many things: genetics, environment, diet, and lifestyle choices. We can't do anything about our genetics, but we can change our beliefs and by changing our beliefs we will automatically change many other options. A positive spirit and a healthy outlook will lead us down a path of supportive choices, whereas a negative outlook keeps us sequestered in a pity party wherein we have a greater tendency to make unhealthy choices.

---

[47] Ibid

One thing leads to another. But there is never a need for *blame*. If illness is anything at all, it is a collection of circumstances that fosters weak soil that then becomes vulnerable to invaders.

We can support the body by doing certain things to maintain its highest functioning capability. The body is best supported by proper nourishment, rest, exercise, and breath. This point is so important that it deserves further exploration.

Proper Nourishment

"You can protect yourself ... through adjustments to diet, exercise and judicious use of vitamins, minerals and herbs."[48]

What we eat plays a huge role in our wellbeing. We want to feed our bodies lightly, greenly and with pure products. In his books, *Health and Healing*, and *Spontaneous Healing*, Andrew Weil suggests that creating and maintaining a strong body and a disease resistant soil requires healthy eating. I have compiled a list of guidelines from several reliable sources over the years. Here are the results of my research:

> *-Reduce overall caloric intake.*
> *(Cut out high fat foods and modify recipes by cutting fat content.)*
> *-Avoid trans fats and saturated fats altogether. Read labels.*
> *- Eat less protein of all kinds.*
> *-Replace animal protein foods with fish and soy foods.*

---

[48] Ibid

*-Cut down on salt. Limit your intake to 1/2
teaspoon per day. be aware of the hidden
sodium in packaged and processed foods.
-Substitute trans fatty acids (margarine,
vegetable shortening, partially hydrogenated
oils, and liquid vegetable oils, polyunsaturated
vegetable oils) with olive oil and a small amount
of canola oil.
-Eat more fruits and vegetables
-Choose fresh over canned or frozen whenever
possible and look for:
Beta = green vegetables and
  Carotene= red/yellow/orange vegetables
-Eat more foods made from whole grains,
cereals, legumes
-Add more dietary fiber: fruits, vegetables, whole
grains.
Insoluble fiber= wheat bran and
Soluble fiber = oat bran.
-Increase consumption of omega-3 fatty acids:
fish, hemp, flax
-Decrease consumption of omega-6 fatty acids:
egg yolks, grain fed meats, particularly   organ
meats, processed foods, and cooking oils
(sunflower, safflower, corn, cottonseed, and
soybean).
-Get rid of high sugar, fructose and sucrose
products, syrups and spreads.*

You can find more information on a proper nutritional
diet by reading Andrew Weil's books, by purchasing
More Ultimate Healing by Bottom Line Publications, or
by doing your own research on the Internet. When you
research the proper diet for you, make sure you look
beyond the slick marketing to evaluate the genuine
benefits of the advice.

Rest

We live in a sleep deprived society. There does not seem to be enough time in a day to accomplish everything on our *to do* list, so we decide that rest is one of those things we can take or leave as our lists dictate. This is erroneous thinking. Rest is a key to creating and maintaining the healthy soil of our bodily environment.
Sleepdex is a nonprofit organization dedicated to collecting and disseminating information about sleep problems.

"Sleep deprivation has become one of the most pervasive health problems facing the United States. It is estimated that people on average now sleep one and a half hours less than people did a century ago.

In a 2002 'Sleep in America' poll of 1,000 adults, nearly a third said that they need at least eight hours to avoid feeling sleepy the next day. However, the respondents responded that they average 6.9 hours of sleep on weeknights and 7.5 on weekend nights. Some experts are even beginning to wonder if widespread sleep deprivation is having an effect on America's brainpower and creativity. A recent U.S. Army study concluded sleep deprivation reduces emotional intelligence and constructive thinking skills. Other short-term consequences include:

>*Increased mortality risk*
>*Decreased daytime alertness. Loss of just one- and one-half hours sleep can result in a 32% reduction in daytime alertness.*
>*Impaired memory and cognitive ability, the ability to think and process information.*

More than double the risk of sustaining an occupational injury.

Impaired immune system.

Long-term consequences can include the following:
High blood pressure
Heart attack
Heart failure
Stroke
Psychiatric problems such as depression and other mood disorders
Mental impairment
Relationship problems with a bed partner
Obesity - (Lack of sleep can cause weight gain by increasing hunger and affecting metabolism; extra weight can cause sleep disorders such as apnea which cause sleep deprivation.)" [49]

Rest is not just sleep, but it is also the time in between our activities. That means work, sports, recreation and anything we concentrate on for long periods of time. The body needs rest. The brain needs rest and diversion. Take breaks, stretch, walk; give your body a chance to settle down from the activity.

Change focus and allow your body to breathe, to reconfigure and to realign. Your body is not a machine. You cannot just screech it to a halt, rotate its tires and go back out onto the fast track. You can try, but you will quickly learn that all of your parts are not equally replaceable, and you will burn out.

---

[49] http://www.sleepdex.org/deficit.htm

Promise yourself that you will take frequent restorative breaks and replenish your resources.

Exercise

In my doctoral health and nutrition courses, one instructor described exercise as being a body massage from the inside out. When we work our muscles, move our bodies and exercise our limbs, we stimulate blood flow, circulate oxygen, refresh hormones and revive our energy levels. When we are inactive we atrophy one ligament, one organ, one system at a time.

The best exercise in the world is walking. Take it from the WebMD site which says:

"Any exercise program should include cardiovascular exercise, which strengthens the heart and burns calories. And walking is something you can do anywhere, anytime, with no equipment other than a good pair of shoes.

It's not just for beginners, either: Even the very fit can get a good workout from walking.

"Doing a brisk walk can burn up to 500 calories per hour," says Robert Gotlin, DO, director of orthopedic and sports rehabilitation at Beth Israel Medical Center in New York. Since it takes 3,500 calories to lose a pound, you could expect to lose a pound for every seven hours you walk, if you did nothing else.

Don't go from the sofa to walking an hour day, though. Richard Cotton, a spokesman for the American Council on Exercise, says beginners should start by walking 5 - 10 minutes at a time, gradually moving up to at least 30 minutes per session. "[50]

Breath

You might not think breathing is that big of a deal. Don't we, after all, do it automatically and naturally? Yes, to remain alive that's true, but to enhance our life, we need to pay attention not just to what we breathe, but also to *how* we breathe. *"You might be amazed to learn that most people don't know that breathing — an act that you do some 20,000 times each day — can deeply influence your health and happiness on many levels. Breathing has been long considered essential for maintaining chi, the life-force energy of Eastern cultural traditions."*

The great Taoist sage Chuang Tzu says, *"...most of us breathe from our throats... real human beings breathe from their heels."* In our bodies breathing oxygenates every cell from our brain to our vital organs. Without sufficient oxygen, our bodies become more susceptible to health problems. Deep breathing raises levels of blood oxygen which promotes cell activity and health. Alternative health icon Dr. Andrew Weil says: *"If I had to limit my advice on healthier living to just one tip, it would be simply to learn how to breathe correctly."*[51]

You would be doing yourself a great favor to take personal training in how to breathe from a knowledgeable teacher. For now, I'm going to give you two ways to increase the breath of health that will allow you to rejuvenate your body, bring oxygen to all organs, and revitalize your blood circulation.

---

[50] http://www.webmd.com/fitness-exercise/guide/7-most-effective-exercises

[51]

http://health.discovery.com/centers/althealth/deepbreath/deepbreathe.html

Sit or stand comfortably. (I would recommend you sit until you get used to practicing correct breathing.) Inhale to fill your lungs. If you feel the first breath in your chest, exhale and then inhale again this time using your abdomen to bring the breath into your body. Let your abdomen expand before the intake of breath. This way your lungs elongate as you draw in air. Try it. Expand your abdomen then allow your breath to fill the lungs, See how easy that is? Do it a few times to get used to the new sequence of actions. Expand your abdomen, breathe in, let your breath fill your lungs on all sides and then gently exhale. You might imagine a flower opening and closing as you breathe in and out.

If you find yourself a little lightheaded, relax. You've probably concentrated too much on the breathing and you've exerted yourself too much. Wait a minute and then try it again. Remember, abdomen first, gentle breath in, expand, and then release your breath. Repeat this activity four times. Rest. Eventually you will be able to sustain this breathing technique for 5-10 minutes, enough to give you a peaceful respite and rejuvenation.

The second process is even more fun. Once you have mastered the previous breathing technique, try this: extend your abdomen, let your breath fill your lungs and now, as if there was a second inhale, allow your breath to fill two invisible lungs around your back. That's right, keep inhaling until all four lungs are filled: two in the front and two in the back, then gently exhale.

Proper breathing is the foundation for all health. If you take a few minutes a day, you will improve rapidly. In any stressful situation you can bring immediate relief by invoking healing breathing techniques. Amazing, life-giving, relaxing and stimulating breath: it's yours for the taking.

Google Dennis Lewis to buy his book: **Ten Secrets of Authentic Breathing**, for more in depth instructions. You can also purchase a CD on breathing techniques by Dr. Andrew Weil.

Howsoever you approach it, begin a regime of breathing and you'll find the rewards incredibly beneficial.

4) *Treat your body like a savings account; store up resources.*

When we think about the body as having, or being, a savings account we begin to see how we need to relate to it. If we store up resources, then we will have what we need when the need arises. We're told by financial experts to create a safety net by having savings equal to six months of our cost of living, just in case we are suddenly out of work. With that savings account, while we look for a new job, we will have the resources we need to go on living.

The same advice applies to the body. If you keep it healthy by feeding it nutritiously, providing the rest it needs, exercising it, and breathing properly, you will store resources in the bank of health. If a challenge comes along you will have the *stored strength* to handle the situation. A friend of mine broke her hip when she was 72, during an ice-skating competition. At the hospital there were several women also in for hip replacement surgery. None of them was in the same great physical condition as my friend.

My friend became the star of the floor. Because she was fit and had strong leg muscles, she recovered in less than half the time of anyone else. She was walking the day after surgery and her recovery took about two and a half weeks instead of the predicted six. Although she was not anticipating needing hip surgery before her slip on the ice, (Did I mention she was *ice skating* at the time of her injury?) her body was prepared for it and handled it with ease. If this preventative method works for hip surgery, imagine what proper care and smart body consciousness would do if a life-threatening disease came knocking on your door. Your health depends on the quality of your soil. Enrich it.

Prevention is the act of taking steps to ward off the unsuspected. It is not creating fear of illness or disease; rather it is protecting yourself from events over which you may have no control. It's like wearing a seat belt as a precaution while driving. Life, by its very nature can be risky. Why not be ready for any and all surprises? Become a storehouse of good health, strong resources and a sturdy constitution. Till your soil regularly.

5) *Cooperate with your body and give it what it needs to serve your life's purpose.*

The body's natural desire is to be well, whole and running smoothly. Our goal is to give it the support it needs to be all of that and fulfill its task. Your body's healing system is always in place, always operative, always ready to work to restore balance when balance is lost; but without proper support its capacity to restore may be inadequate for a required task.

We enrich our soil by employing all of the methods we have just discussed. We can also call upon our inner healer for additional guidance and direction. *"Anyone who comes to see healing as an innate capacity of the body rather than something to be sought outside it, will gain greater power over the fluctuations of health and illness. Anyone who recognizes the importance of mind and belief in determining responses to treatments will be able to make better sense of past interactions with medical practitioners and better decisions about future ones."* [52]

Exercise

There are questions which we can pose that will give us further insight into ways in which we can cooperate with our bodies. You may want to use your pendulum for guidance if the answers don't come easily.

At this moment does my body require more:

> Rest? (Getting away from it all, more sleep, peace, quiet).
> Better Nutrition? (A different diet?)
> Exercise? (Movement?)
> Breath? (Breathing exercises, a breath of fresh air, a change of climate?)

---

[52] Andrew Weil, *Spontaneous Healing*

Refer to the pendulum chart in Chapter Five for more ideas.

When you begin to cooperate in the healing process you will discover that your body, mind and heart are already way ahead of you. Your job in this Third Act is to research all of the possibilities for healing that your body might require; to believe in the power of healing and your innate ability to heal; and to allow your heart to guide you through the rocky terrain of past disappointments into the possibilities of a fantastic future.

Chapter Seven

The Final Act: Supreme Healing

"No longer is God to be found in the clouds or burning bush. The curtain secluding the holy of holies has been torn in half; healing is within waiting to be released."
Author

The final scene in the Three Act play synthesizes all of the previous action and dialog and creates a closing moment that provides the raison d'être of the play. This is the fulcrum point, the moment of revelation and solution. Everything that has come before is shown to be meaningful and to have purpose, all of the loose ends are wrapped up and the instant of truth is revealed. All that remains is for the final curtain to fall and for the audience to express its appreciation in appropriate applause.

At this point in *Supreme Healing* we have experienced our first Three Acts: Conviction, Connection and Cooperation. In the first act, Conviction, we studied the depth and the power of the main character, Spirit. We learned how to relate to, and believe in, Its unlimited wisdom and power. In the second act, Connection, we moved deeper into our awareness of that Power and we not only related to the Power, but we connected to it.

We became one with God, acknowledging that we are the same mind, the same wisdom; and that Spirit's power is our own. In the third act, Cooperation, we have learned how to support what we have discovered and to follow the inner wisdom we have accrued. We have become the intuitive and the artist, engaging in the necessary steps to encourage our inner healer into manifestation. Now the final scene in the last act gives us the last word and concludes our play.

Your inner wisdom has led you to the Grace of healing. You have taken the time to listen to the inner voice that knows everything you need to know to coach healing from dormancy into activity. You have touched on a variety of channels where your healing could be supported and now we arrive at the final moment, the icing on the cake and the grand finale of our healing.

In the words of Carolyn Myss, *"The fact is that the body and the mind alone cannot disintegrate an army of cancer cells that have invaded multiple organs, whereas that highly refined spiritual substance that I refer to as grace, combined with the resources of the heart and the mind can ascend to mystical heights."*[53]

You now know how to stage your healing. You have acquired an understanding of the healing process and stocked your mind with the beliefs that lead to unlocking your inner artist and healer.
We are now ready for the final scene. Ultimately everything has led up to this and all of the understanding, knowledge and experiences of the preceding acts can now be brought together to reveal the moment of truth for which we have been preparing. It is time for the grand finale.

---

[53] Carolyn Myss, *Defying Gravity*

The spiritual process that you are about to embark upon to create your *Supreme Healing* is called: *Cooking the Egg*. The process is simple, but the outcome is powerful.

There are three steps to our *cooking* process. The terms are familiar, but this last scene of Act Three is where the *magic* happens, and it results in the creation of something far greater than the sum of its parts. The invisible infuses the visible and healing results.

Cooking the Egg:

Step One: Conviction

Assemble the materials in your mind: you will need a pan of water, an egg and a stove.   The water represents the Power of the Almighty; the egg holds the creative thought in your mind (the healing you see for yourself) and the stove is your passion. When you are ready to begin, in your mind's eye, place the water on the stove and hold the egg in your hand.

Look deeply into the water. This is the Presence of God. Water has a fluid power; it takes all shapes and forms. Water surrounds you in the form of air, it is in the earth beneath you, and it is in you as 70% of your substance. Feel the Presence of God as the   water. Feel it inside of you and all around you. Feel that oneness and sense at the deepest level as you and the water flow in and through one another. Become as a sponge to the water, let it circulate through every pore. Allow your awareness to become the conviction that you are one with the Power and the Wisdom and the Knowledge that God is All there is and is here, now, within the water, within you. Continue to focus on the water until you are completely convinced you are united with it. In your mind touch the water and feel that contact at the core of your being. You share the creative power of the Universe and you are a co-creator with the Divine.

Inseparable, integrated, peaceful and potent; you can feel the Power and the Presence of God in every cell of your body. Know that there is nothing this Power as you cannot accomplish.

Step Two: Connection

Now, shift your attention from the water to the egg that you hold in your hand. The egg   is neutral. With your thoughts impress into the egg the picture of the condition or   circumstance that you want to create. Picture the ideal.

See yourself relieved of any previous limitation. Picture yourself completely healed. You are creating a new vision for your life, a vision that is healed, whole and free of any past, undesired condition. Make your vision strong, clear and as detailed as you can. Your new vision dissolves any condition or thing that is not exactly as you see it. Know that all opposition falls away and perfection arises like a Phoenix from the ashes. Believe that Divine Power supports you in your vision of wholeness and brings it into manifestation.

See your desired state, add anything else you need to complete it. Hold the picture firmly in your mind; impress that image into the center of the egg. Allow the substance of the egg to absorb your mental picture, merging it fully into itself.

When you have impressed your thoughts into the egg, turn up the flame under the water. Feel the heat rising and watch as the fire unleashes the power within the water and brings it to a boil. This is the Power of God in action, the Power that works for you, as you and through you. This Creative Force bubbles up all around you with undeniable might and vigor. This Force of Creation animates Life itself.

Turn the power up again and increase the energy. Feel the water rise to a rolling boil. See the Power reflected in the water as the heat increases. Now hold that image of the Power of Creation unleashed, in your mind and feel it resonate all the way down to your toes. Connect to the Power. Feel the power of the now boiling water deep inside your being.

Step Three: Cooperation

When the water reaches the intensity of a full rolling boil, feel that rumble in your bones. Now it is time to place the egg into the water. The egg holds your vision of wholeness. With absolute confidence, release the egg into the powerfully boiling water and watch as the water accepts it, wraps itself around it and welcomes it enthusiastically. Know with absolute certainty that the boiling water now cooks this egg, making what is contained within it solid and real. The water can do nothing else but cook your egg. You have done your part. Now, God takes over. Turn the flame up under the water one more time. With the passion in your heart and the conviction of your soul, increase the heat to intensify the boiling action. The egg dances freely in this amazing energy, as it cooks solid in the water of Divine Action. In your mind, remain united with the water as it cooks the egg perfectly into the form of your vision. See your healed condition in full, vivid, saturated living color. Hold that picture full screen in your mind.

When the Egg is cooked, you are healed. Your thought has become your reality, and nothing can prevent this from being so. As easily as the water of Divine Supply receives your egg and cooks it according to your mental picture, so too becomes the physical manifestation of your healing.

Believe with all your heart that in this moment you are healed. Take a moment to thank this incredible power and the Essence within you which allows this Act of Creation to turn your egg from a thought into manifest reality. Accept this as Truth and let it be so.

Chapter Eight

Encore

*"Always be joyful, no matter what you are... Every day
we must deliberately induce in ourselves a buoyant,
exuberant attitude toward life; in this manner, we will
gradually become receptive to the subtle mysteries
around us. And, if no inspired moments seem to come,
we should act as though we have them anyway."*
Rabbi Nachman

Do not be discouraged if healing doesn't seem to occur
instantly. Every part of life has its distinct rhythm.
Healing can happen in an instant, or it can take place
over a lifetime. Your job is to stay convinced, remain
connected, and continue to cooperate. There are times
when you may require extra courage; summon it. There
may be times when you need extra help; ask for it. As
long as you remain committed to your healing process
you will attract exactly what is required to accomplish
the task.

If anyone asks you what they can do to help, have a list
ready. Friends and family love to help you if they are
given specific directions. When my mother passed
away it was during a very difficult and busy time of my
life. I was surrounded by deadlines. Friends asked me
what they could do to help. I took their offers seriously. I
made a list of everything that had to be accomplished,
organized, researched, and ordered.

Each friend tackled his or her assignment with energy and competence. The list contained requests for everything from out of state contacts for dumpsters, handy men, caterers, realtors, appraisers, movers and printers. Somehow they all found the time and resources to help me, while I was dealing with my loss and handling multiple crises at work. It was an awesome lesson and I was grateful for all their help. I could not have done it without them.

What kind of help do you need in your healing process:

>Do you need help with daily household chores or animal care?
>Do you need help researching your condition?
>Do you need referrals to health practitioners, doctors, specialists?
>Do you need to bounce ideas off of someone?
>Do you need understanding?
>Do you need transportation ?
>Do you need to research facilities or treatments?
>Do you need to locate chat rooms or online support?

Remember we are not alone in this human experience. If you feel like you are inconveniencing someone, change your mind and allow them the honor of helping you. One of the most beautiful qualities about our humanity is that we all enjoy being of value. Ask for help when you need it.

When you have the Conviction that God is all there is, the real Source of healing; when you have made a deep and personal Connection with that Power; and when you have explored every possibility to improve your condition through Cooperation, have accepted the outcome, and are living from your heart center, you have achieved *Supreme Healing*. Congratulations.

Everyone alive can achieve this level of healing. As long as there is breath in your body, you can heal. Always remember your Inner Violet, she's with you all the time.

I know and believe this from experience. I have healed from many physical and emotional challenges and I support and encourage you to do the same. I wrote this book for you, and as a tribute to Violet, with all my love.

Secrets of Healing

The Lessons from Squirrels: *Love and Peanuts*

"Healing is a matter of time, but it is sometimes also a matter of opportunity." Hippocrates

I want to share with you a little story that illustrates the natural and practical application of the properties of healing and how I watched them in action in my own back yard, quite by accident. This incident inspired me to write this book and my teachers, this time, were tree squirrels.

We have four squirrels that are part of the outdoor extended family in our forest. In addition to the deer, the woodpeckers, the moonlit stealthy raccoons, the blue jays, the occasional red fox and the local crows, we have four squirrels who have taken up residency, close enough to hear a peanut drop, should such an incident occur, on the back deck.

It began innocently enough when a lone squirrel showed up at the back door, stood on his hind legs, and showed us his red, raw, burnt underbelly. When two compassionate, caring, nurturing individuals see a small creature in distress, pain and need, it took every ounce of courage and conviction not to open the screen door and welcome the little fella in with open arms.

Thoughts raced through my mind: *"Should I treat him with hydrogen peroxide to cleanse the wounds? Should I plaster his body with Neosporin? Should we make a little bed for him and cover him while we minister to his every want and need? Should I bottle feed him? Would he nap when we told him to? Will he take the bus to school? How could we help?"* Immediately, I pictured a healing room for him outfitted with a squirrel-sized bed, tiny bandages, a bowl of water on a silver platter for him, and soothing strokes for his little grey furry head.

He rose up on his back legs a second time to display the results of his encounter with a live wire, or two, and our hearts broke for him. *"Squirrels: what do they like to eat?"* I assaulted the crevices of my brain to shake loose any stored information on the diets of squirrels. *"Nuts"* popped into the middle of my mind. *"Nut, nuts, Nuts."* I tore through every kitchen cabinet and found a bag of pine nuts. Yes. Pine nuts it was! I crept outside with a bowl of pine nuts, and sure enough, in record time he was munching and chomping and filling his scorched body with this imported delicacy.

When he finished all of the pine nuts, he leapt up onto the railing and promptly fell asleep on the warm wood. Long after the sun made its final exit from the forest that evening, he was on my mind. I planned many feats of rescue so I might abscond with him and take him to a vet for care. I thought of a peanut-butter laced humane trap, a butterfly net, cornering him with a blanket and swooping him up for transport over my shoulder as a wiggling bundle of reluctant nature. I didn't own a trap, the only net I had was for a long-since-departed fish tank, and the only blanket I could think of was a purple hand knitted throw from the sofa. I slept fitfully that night.

The next morning, he returned. I raided the freezer in the garage and found slivered almonds, a few more pine nuts, some limp pistachios and a few outdated walnuts from holiday baking. I made a mixture of the nuts and poured a helping *into his dish*. The munching commenced.

It took everything I had in my spiritual warehouse not to "help" the squirrel heal. He had bravely shown us his injuries and we had responded thinking, at first, that we needed to *do* something to help him out of his predicament. I took myself by the scruff of my neck, shook myself and said, *"Let the squirrel alone. He is perfectly capable of healing. You do not need to DO anything. Pray for him. Shower him with Conviction and love. Let that little being realize his own co-creation and just BE there for him."* I fought with myself, *"But I could help him,"* I thought, *"I could fix him. I have healing ointments and a car. I could take him places and he will get better."*

But something stronger fought back. *"Leave him do what he needs to do. Just believe in him."* In that instant I realized that I could DO more good for him by knowing what was in my heart, and summoning the patience to allow him his own experience of whatever his healing process needed to be. At first it was a torturously difficult decision. It's very hard to watch an innocent being suffer, especially when I believed I had the tools of healing in my medicine cabinet. This squirrel had shown me his physical damage, but he was teaching me how Spirit really heals. All I had to do was watch and learn. I decided that I would both *DO* and *BE* for him. The DOing came in the form of research. The BEing came later. I Googled *"squirrel diet"* and found the following:

"*The gray squirrel's diet consists of nuts, seeds and fruit. It will eat bird eggs, bugs, and even an animal carcass if there is no other food source available.*"

"*Yikes,*" I thought to myself, "*I don't want this little guy eating a carcass, so I'll go get him some peanuts.*" Fortunately, one of the larger membership stores carries giant bags of unsalted peanuts for the health aware.

What a discovery. I raced home with my *find* and proceeded to fill Owie Guy's dish with fresh peanuts. Hooray! He showed up and dove into them like the ravenous rodent he was.

We named him *Owie Guy* because, by now, another squirrel had shown up, (I suppose from having smelled the wafting of fresh peanuts across the pine limbs) and was beckoned to the deck like a mesmerized cobra. Two squirrels, no waiting. We named the first visitor, Owie Guy so we could tell them apart, assuming that it mattered.

Additional Internet search enlightened me further: "*The gray squirrel requires some salt in its diet and may find this salt in the soil along roads where snow and ice may have been*". Oh No! I had purchased the *unsalted* peanuts thinking these to be the best and the healthiest for the squirrel, but now it appeared I may be depriving him. Poor little dude, he must be *dying* for some salt. Keys in the ignition and back to the store I went. This time for a bag of the salted peanuts to mix with the unsalted so Owie Guy didn't have to lick the pavement or be bothered by having to travel to the mountains to look for icy roads.

Returning once again to the Internet, I read: *"Squirrels chew on tree branches to sharpen and clean their teeth. That's why you may see many small branches on the ground around large trees. They will also chew on power lines for the same reason; this has caused many major power outages throughout the country."*

Okay, so that's what happened. It was the chewing thing on the power lines that got him in trouble. I pictured, "Scurry, scurry, scurry, Chomp, chomp, tszzzzt! YOWZAH!" Or a scenario close to that.

"A squirrel's brain is about the size of a walnut." Well, that makes sense. If he had a brain the size of an avocado pit, maybe he wouldn't bite live power lines. I don't know. Maybe size doesn't matter; just how you *use* what you've got, brain-wise.

Every day, twice a day, without fail, Owie Guy showed up, ate his peanuts and then took his healing nap on the sun-warmed railing. Each visit he stood outside the screen door, only inches away from us, and showed us how his underside was coming along. We continued to tell him how beautiful he was, how much we loved him and how nicely his fur was growing in. Apparently, he thought so, too.

More information: *"The average adult squirrel needs to eat about a pound of food a week to maintain an active life."*

The arrival of the second squirrel was putting a big dent in the original peanut supply. Back to the store I went for another purchase of *both* varieties of peanuts. That errand led to another in which I purchased a large, sealable storage container to hold the mix of the salted and unsalted peanuts. We needed squirrel food to be fresh and handy at all times, didn't we?

Owie Guy had become so friendly, (and more precise in his timing than Big Ben) that he was a solid fixture at the back door at 7:15 every morning. If, by some chance, the household wanted to sleep until the languid hour of 8:00 am, Owie Guy would scamper outside the bedroom window, jump up and down, and make such a fuss that it was impossible to sleep. "*There must be something very healing in those peanuts, as he's awfully frisky for someone as hurt as he looks,*" we muttered as we stumbled out of bed towards the kitchen to dole out his shell-covered medicine.

In a matter of a few days, the second squirrel had become a regular, and took to climbing atop the outside water bottle when peanut service was not as timely as desired. Noticing a piece of this one's right ear missing, he was dubbed *Clipper* because something or someone had indeed clipped his ear and left a permanent indentation. Clipper and Owie Guy were quite a pair.

It was not long before existence of the peanut express had been communicated throughout the forest. Many came to sample, but only a few remained as boarders. Next on the scene was *Poodle Tail* so named because of an encounter, we believed with another power line, which took most of the fur off his tail from the heinie up, but left a round poof at the end, hence the name Poodle Tail.

Now there were three. An occasional stranger would show up from time to time, but rarely stayed for more than a quick hors d'oeuvre. Perhaps they were frightened away by Clipper's sometimes assertive chasing. The smart ones snuck in for a peanut while Clipper was off on a romp after a greedy blue jay or an interested crow. The fourth squirrel arrived with one blind eye. Helen joined the motley crew.

The cats that live in our house have become extremely fond of the squirrels too. The alpha male assertively comes to remind either one of us that the peanut supply needs to be enhanced as there are hungry squirrels impatiently in need of a snack. Many tails thump when the supply diminishes. The squirrels are so friendly now we have been tempted to hand feed them their peanuts. Fortunately, the Internet advises against unnatural or overly mano-friendly interactions:

The most common type of squirrel bite is a result of feeding a squirrel by hand. Never hold the food between your fingers; chances are very good you will be bitten. A squirrel's eyes are always looking for predators and they rarely focus on what they are eating.[54] Good to know.

As Owie Guy transformed into *Wowie Guy*, the lesson for me became the awareness of allowing the inner healer to surface. So too, the caution to not overdo it was welcome enlightenment.
It's been a few months now since I wanted to build a bed for the injured squirrel. He is now fully recovered, faithfully on time for feedings, and even brought his baby to visit. The squirrel family has increased and multiplied.

---

[54] http://www.squirrels.org/facts.html

Wowie Guy, Clipper, Poodle Tail , Helen and now the baby, which we have aptly named *Peanut,* are regulars. We have no clue whose child Peanut actually is, but we're happy to see them all and would like to think it's Wowie Guy's. Peanut is young, beautiful and bright eyed with a bushy tail. He (or she) is pristine. There isn't a mark on him or her, nary a scar nor a blemish. Hard knocks have not entered the baby's lexicon of experience yet.

He or she lives in the protected aura of youth, untouched by life or power lines. If you wanted a candidate for a squirrel poster, this would be your ideal. I love the idea that Peanut is Wowie's baby and he brought his progeny to show us the full extent of his turnaround. I like to think that, but it really doesn't matter.

I would love to take credit for *the healing peanuts,* but I know better. All we did was provide the atmosphere for Wowie Guy to heal himself.

We became his supply of food, so he could attend to the business of allowing his inner healer to take the natural path to full recovery. We stayed out of his way, put our personal agendas aside and loved him with all our hearts, even though our egos craved to do more. The lesson for me is that we did what we were called to do for him, as his assistants to his self-healing.

We were all in it together: us, Wowie Guy and God. He may have easily found others to attend to his food supply needs, but he chose us. We were invited to witness his process, and the rewards of his inner strength. If he didn't believe, at his core level, even with his walnut sized brain, that he could heal, or at least if he wasn't open to healing, he wouldn't have. His squirrel consciousness was so high that it probably never occurred to him that he would not heal. As a result, he did. Everything unfolded perfectly for him to support his recovery and regrowth.

For as long as I am asked to, I will provide him with what he requires. He became my teacher and a wise conduit for me to learn the lesson of staying out of the way while something bigger works. Peanuts and love were all that was required of me.

The web article left me with one last squirrel fact: *"The squirrel's erratic path while crossing a street is an attempt to confuse the oncoming vehicle... thereby causing it to change direction. This is obliviously the squirrels biggest, and often last mistake."* Okay, now I'm calling a meeting! *"Wowie Guy, Clipper, Poodle Tail, Helen, Peanut....come here, now. Momma wants to talk to you!"*[55] [56]

---

[55] http://www.squirrels.org/facts.html

[56] After more research we realized that squirrels require more than peanuts to be healthy. Before you write letter of protest please be aware we have added the appropriate foods to their diet along with calcium supplements.

I leave you with one last question: What is your *healing peanut?* And, who might assist you in obtaining it? What is it that will take you from the pain and suffering you feel today into a healed state?

I hope you have gained a clearer perspective on how to activate your own inner healer and have learned a tool or two for accomplishing your personal and *Supreme Healing*.

Appendix

Excerpts from: FactMonster
http://www.factmonster.com/ipka/.html . For more
details and further information go to their site.

Your Body's Systems[57]
Circulatory System
The circulatory system is the body's transport system. It
is made up of a group of organs that transport blood
throughout the body. The heart pumps the blood and
the **arteries** and **veins** transport it. Oxygen-rich blood
leaves the left side of the heart and enters the biggest
artery, called the **aorta**. Veins carry waste products
away from cells and bring blood back to the heart,
which pumps it to the lungs to pick up oxygen and
eliminate waste carbon dioxide.

Digestive System
The digestive system is made up of organs that break
down food into protein, vitamins, minerals,
carbohydrates, and fats, which the body needs for
energy, growth, and repair. The excess food that the
body doesn't need or can't digest is turned into waste
and is eliminated from the body.

Endocrine System

---

[57] "http://www.factmonster.com/ipka/.html." Fact
Monster.
© 2000–2007 Pearson Education, publishing as Fact
Monster.
15 Jul. 2010
<http://www.factmonster.com/ipka/A0774536.html>.

The endocrine system is made up of a group of glands that produce the body's long-distance messengers, or hormones. Hormones are chemicals that control body functions, such as metabolism, growth, and sexual development. The glands, which include the pituitary gland, thyroid gland, parathyroid glands, adrenal glands, thymus gland, pineal body, pancreas, ovaries, and testes, release hormones directly into the bloodstream, which transports the hormones to organs and tissues throughout the body.

Immune System
The immune system is our body's defense system against infections and diseases. Organs, tissues, cells, and cell products work together to respond to dangerous organisms (like viruses or bacteria) and substances that may enter the body from the environment. There are three types of response systems in the immune system: the anatomic response, the inflammatory response, and the immune response.

- The **anatomic response** physically prevents threatening substances from entering your body. Examples of the anatomic system include the mucous membranes and the skin. If substances do get by, the inflammatory response goes on attack.
- The **inflammatory system** works by excreting the invaders from your body. Sneezing, runny noses, and fever are examples of the inflammatory system at work. Sometimes, even though you don't feel well while it's happening, your body is fighting illness.
- When the inflammatory response fails, the **immune response** goes to work. This is the central part of the immune system and is made up of white blood cells, which fight infection by gobbling up antigens.

Lymphatic System

The lymphatic system is also a defense system for the body. It filters out organisms that cause disease, produces white blood cells, and generates disease-fighting antibodies. It also distributes fluids and nutrients in the body and drains excess fluids and protein so that tissues do not swell. The lymphatic system is made up of a network of vessels that help circulate body fluids. These vessels carry excess fluid away from the spaces between tissues and organs and return it to the bloodstream.

Muscular System

The muscular system is made up of tissues that work with the skeletal system to control movement of the body. Some muscles—like the ones in your arms and legs—are voluntary, meaning that you decide when to move them. Other muscles, like the ones in your stomach, heart, intestines and other organs, are involuntary. This means that they are controlled automatically by the nervous system and hormones— you often don't even realize they're at work.

Nervous System

The nervous system is made up of the brain, the spinal cord, and nerves. One of the most important systems in your body, the nervous system is your body's control system. It sends, receives, and processes nerve impulses throughout the body. These nerve impulses tell your muscles and organs what to do and how to respond to the environment. There are three parts of your nervous system that work together:

- The **central nervous system** consists of the brain and spinal cord. It sends out nerve impulses and analyzes information from the sense organs, which tell your brain about things you see, hear, smell, taste and feel.
- The **peripheral nervous system** includes the craniospinal nerves that branch off from the brain and the spinal cord. It carries the nerve impulses from the central nervous system to the muscles and glands.
- The **autonomic nervous system** regulates involuntary action, such as heartbeat and digestion.

Reproductive System

The reproductive system allows humans to produce children. Sperm from the male fertilizes the female's egg, or ovum, in the fallopian tube. The fertilized egg travels from the fallopian tube to the uterus, where the fetus develops over a period of nine months.

Respiratory System

The respiratory system brings air into the body and removes carbon dioxide. It includes the nose, trachea, and lungs. When you breathe in, air enters your nose or mouth and goes down a long tube called the trachea. Oxygen follows this path and passes through the walls of the air sacs and blood vessels and enters the blood stream. At the same time, carbon dioxide passes into the lungs and is exhaled.

Skeletal System

The skeletal system is made up of bones, ligaments and tendons. It shapes the body and protects organs.

The skeletal system works with the muscular system to help the body move. Marrow, which is the soft, fatty tissue which produces red blood cells, many white blood cells, and other immune system cells, is found inside bones.

Urinary System
The urinary system eliminates waste from the body, in the form of urine. The kidneys remove waste from the blood. The waste combines with water to form urine.

Source Notes

Invisible Supply, Joel. S. Goldsmith
The Intelligent Heart, David McArthur & Bruce McArthur
Health & Healing, Andrew Weil M.D.
Keys to Health, Eric A. Mein M. D.
Spontaneous Healing, Andrew Weil, M.D.
Becoming God(s), Marlene Morris D.D.
www.ReleventSpirituality.com
Opus Lux, Christa Rae Pacheco   www.OpusLux.com
Kahuna Healing, Serge King
The Three Sisters of the Tao, Terah Kathryn Collins
Your Mind: The Owner's Manual, Linda Joy Rose
The Science of Mind, Ernest Holmes
Defying Gravity, Carolyn Myss
Power Versus Force, David Hawkins
The Eye of the I, David Hawkins
Beyond Words and Thoughts, Joel Goldsmith
More Ultimate Healing, Bottom Line Publications

More books by

_____

kac young, PhD, ND. DCH, RScM

Discover Your Spiritual Genius
A compendium of helpful shortcuts for your spiritual development. This is the beginner's guide to knowing it all. You need this book if you're feeling down in the dumps or if your life isn't working the way you want it to. If you read and follow this advice life will take on a new meaning, you will be on top of your game, in charge of your life, happier, and more fulfilled.

Feng Shui, the Easy Way
The ancient art from China that can change your life overnight. This is a shortcut to proven Feng Shui principles and practices which can create immediate results in your life. Harmonize your life by balancing the "stuff" in it. It's easier than you think. The results are life-altering for the good.

Dancing With the Moon
Learn how to use the natural energies of the lunar forces to orchestrate your life, your emotions and to create a deeper experience of living life at its fullest measure. Dancing With the Moon is easy to learn and simple to use. You will be enriched daily with this process. There is nothing more healing than living in rhythm with the lunar phases.

Chart Your Course - online only
http://chartyourcourse12.com/

Create the year you want and fulfill your dreams by working with the energies of the stars and the planets. You can create the life you have always wanted by following these 12 simple steps to harness the cosmic energies that are just out there waiting for you. It's a process that will change your inner life and manifest what you truly want to have in your outer life.

The Healing Art of Essential Oils
A wonderful introduction to the art of using essential oils with lots of recipes and profiles for 50 oils. Brilliant book for the beginner or advanced user. Highly recommended by experts.

The Art of Healing with Crystals, a wonderful book that explains all about crystal energies and how you can use them to help yourself emotionally, physically and spiritually.

The One Minute Cat Manager, Sixty Seconds to Shangri-La. This book is a wonderful romp through cat companionship and shows you how you can manage a cat no matter how busy you are with these 60 second ideas. Delightful stories and entertaining drawings make this book a must-have. Bedtime stories for cats will delight you and kitty. Practical information will help you understand your cat and deepen your bond.

Natural Healing for Cats Combining Bach Flower Remedies and Behavioral Therapy, The gentle way to help your feline friends. This book outlines which Bach Flower Remedy is appropriate for what feline condition. It's a force-free way to assist cats and change unwanted behaviors. Use this gentle way to help your cats heal, cope and adjust to life with humans.

Gold Mind is a book about managing your finances, learning about money management and creating your personal wealth one paycheck at a time. This book will change your thinking about money and help you increase your prosperity. Highly recommended by financial experts.

Supreme Healing is a Master guideline to healing. No matter what you want to heal in body, mind or spirit, you can use this book as your ladder to success. It contains all the thinking and processes you'll ever need to heal yourself.

The Ultimate Guide to Crystals for Healing and Beyond. This is the intermediate book on crystal healing, techniques and combinations with essential oils, crystals, chakras, astrology, archetypes and the 12 Laws of Karma for deep and effective healing. If you want to heal yourself or are a healer, this book is a must-have for your practice and library.

The Quick Guide to Bach Flower Remedies. If you've ever wondered how Bach Flowers work, you need this book. It is designed to give you a quick, thorough and easy reference for the use and effectiveness of Bach Flowers. You can heal by just looking at the paintings of each flower. It is exquisite and full of vibrational healing ideas and techniques. Purchase at: https://www.kacyoung.com/product/bach-flower-remedies/   The book is NOT available on Amazon

VISIT www.kacyoung.com for more information on each book.

Private consultation is available for any and all of these subjects: PO Box 6102, Ventura ,CA. 93003 or